MEDICINE
UNDER ATTACK

AND OTHER ESSAYS

CLYDE W. JOHNSON M.D.

Library of Congress Control Number:		2013902573
ISBN:	Hardcover	978-1-4797-9346-4
	Softcover	978-1-4797-9345-7
	Ebook	978-1-4797-9347-1

This book was printed in the United States of America.

Rev. date: 2/21/2013

To order additional copies of this book, contact:
Xlibris Corporation
1-888-795-4274
www.Xlibris.com
Orders@Xlibris.com

ALSO AVAILABLE

AUTOBIOGRAPHY OF CLYDE W. JOHNSON, MD

THE END
of an
ERA

Clyde W. Johnson, MD

Thank you to Daniele Washburn, MBA, for her technical assistance in producing this book.

PART I

CHAPTER I

This book is about my experiences, observations, and opinions. We are all entitled to our own opinions, and this is mine. I'm sure there are those who see things differently and have different opinions.

I graduated from Indiana University in 1961, before Medicare or Medicaid was law. Since most young men were required to serve some time in the military service at that time, I had been in ROTC at Purdue for four years prior to going to medical school. So I was required to go on active duty and chose to do a rotating internship in the army and then serve my required two years more of active duty. I therefore had an introduction to government-controlled medical care for three years and decided I didn't want to continue in that environment.

I was released from active duty in the spring of 1964 as the Vietnam War was escalating. Since I had a wife and four children to support, I didn't want to be recalled to active duty. I resigned my commission and found a position in a small town in Idaho to live and practice family medicine. Council, Idaho, had one doctor, Dr. E., and a twenty-bed hospital for a town of eight hundred, a county of three thousand, and a few small communities outside the county not served by another doctor. I joined Dr. E. for a monthly stipend of $1,000. That was more than I was receiving as an army medical officer; however, in the army, I also had a house provided.

For several years, there had been a faction complaining about the high cost of medical care in the United States. That included many newspapers, magazines, and especially politicians and other government spokesmen. I think also many businesses wanted the government involved in medical care so the businesses could shift the cost of medical insurance for their employees to the government in the mistaken thought that the cost would be less, never recognizing that when government is involved, the cost goes up.

At that time in 1964, our charge for a routine office visit was $4. Complete obstetrics care—including all prenatal, delivery, postpartum care to six weeks, and newborn care to six weeks—was $75. A circumcision, if requested, was $5 extra but might be cancelled if the family was poor, a common circumstance in rural Idaho. An appendectomy was also $75. I don't know how much the hospital charged for those services, but it was about the same amount. I do know the daily room rates at that time. A private room was $19, and a double room was $21. Medicare came into being in 1964. When I left Idaho in 1967, our charges for complete obstetric care was $100, and for an appendectomy, it was also $100. The hospital's charges had gone up to $25 for a double room and $27 for a private room.

I want to briefly describe the type of medicine we provided in those days in Idaho. We had a main office in Council with an x-ray and a small lab, which was staffed by one of us doctors, a nurse, and a receptionist / billing clerk five days a week. We also had three outlying clinics in three small communities, each about twenty-five miles up or down the mountains from Council. Those towns were Midvale, New Meadows, and Riggins. The Midvale office also served the small town of Cambridge, which was nearby. Riggins was a small town next to the Salmon

River. We took turns manning these clinics half a day twice a week with a part-time nurse and one of us doctors. The nurses lived in the communities we served, but the doctors drove there each time. I did this traveling for the three years I was in Idaho and never was reimbursed for my gas to do the traveling by the medical partnership, nor did I deduct the expense from my taxes. I never even thought of it at the time. I was too busy, I suppose, or was caught up in my sense of professional responsibilities.

Medicaid was not yet implemented while I was in Idaho, but there was, nevertheless, welfare for the poor and medical care for those on welfare. The county supervisors designated those deserving of welfare and paid our medical partnership $100 a month to provide any and all medical care a welfare recipient needed. After I left Idaho, I heard the county raised their payment to the only doctor left to $1,000 a month.

I left my medical practice in Idaho in 1967 largely because it was difficult to earn enough money to support and educate my five children. The people were great on the surface but were not very sophisticated about the modern world. They frequently complained about even our modest charges, then went long distances to another doctor for a physical exam or other service that we could do locally.

Medical care wasn't the only thing not understood. For example, there was lots of complaining about "Californians" buying up the land and ranches for prices the locals thought were exorbitant and couldn't afford. Also, I saw many times local people would go to Boise ninety miles away to stock up on groceries instead of buying from the local grocery store, never realizing they might put the local store out of business.

CHAPTER 2

I joined a surgeon in Southern California to do family medicine after leaving Idaho. Soon after moving to California, I met all the requirements for board certification and did so for my own gratification and to meet some of the insurance companies' requirements for participation. I stayed in that partnership for thirty years and had a large patient following. The move to California was a real eye-opener as far as seeing the direction medical care was going. In spite of what I'm writing about in the rest of this book, I had a great career in medicine and wouldn't have wanted to do anything else in my lifetime. My career was during the golden era of medicine when tremendous advances in medicine and medical technology were implemented. I had a part in that by constant study to keep current for my patient's benefit. I'm pleased to have had a satisfying and rewarding professional career.

Sometime in the 1960s, California had changed all doctors of osteopathy to doctors of medicine simply by the legislature passing a law. The idea was to eliminate the perception that there were two levels of medical care in California, the lower quality being the osteopaths. The plan was to upgrade the schools of osteopathy to medical schools. The upgrade plan was good, but what about the already trained osteopaths that were trained at the possibly lower-quality schools? This move by the government was one of the first government actions that I observed that I thought lowered the quality of medical care. Many of the former osteopaths that I knew went to many continuing medical education classes to upgrade their skills, so there was some benefit to the state's action. I applaud those doctors of osteopathy as I think their action helped keep the quality of medical care in California at an acceptable level for many years.

Some years later, Governor Jerry Brown proposed and pushed for lower-level health care workers after he went on a trip to China where he saw health care workers providing care in rural areas at a very low cost. He and the Chinese called them barefoot doctors. Because of this push by Governor Brown and others, we now have less-trained people (nurse practitioners and physicians' assistants) treating many of us. This move to less training is supposed to cut the cost of medical care. I think it only saved money for the various government agencies and for many insurance companies. After all, if you pay someone less, there is more profit for the insurance company. I'm not sure at all that paying the lower-level providers less money is less expensive in the long run or that they deserve less for what they do. As proof of that, look at the continuing complaints of the cost of medical care many years after implementing the physicians' assistant and nurse practitioner programs.

In the late sixties and early seventies, Senator Ted Kennedy conducted "hearings" around the country about poor and/or expensive medical care. Kennedy was chairman of a health care committee. Some of those hearings were in the Los Angeles area. What I heard were false or exaggerated allegations of wrongdoings, overcharging, and other claims to blame doctors and other health professionals for things they didn't do so the government should take over the management of all health care to stop these wrongdoings and inefficiencies.

During President Kennedy's term in office, there was

a law passed allowing foreign-trained medical doctors to come to the United States for advanced training and then stay in the United States permanently. I can personally attest to this as my Filipino partner, Dr. Tan, had a plaster bust of President Kennedy in his office to celebrate the action allowing Dr. Tan and many others of my acquaintance to practice medicine in this country. The stated purpose at the time the measure was implemented was to alleviate the "doctor shortage" and to have an adequate supply of doctors so the cost of medical care would be controlled. Here we are, fifty years later, still importing foreign-trained doctors for the "doctor shortage" and complaining of even much higher medical care costs. I think we should be training our own children to be physicians instead of importing them.

Let's look at that issue for a moment. The doctors getting their medical school training in a foreign country must get further training in the United States by taking a residency in a specialty to be upgraded to stay in the United States to practice medicine. Over the past fifty years, there has been a massive immigration of doctors to this country, and almost all of them are in some type of specialty other than general practice. With a huge number of these specialist and super specialists, there is pressure to have any illness you might have treated by a specialist even if a family doctor or a general practitioner could treat it as well or better. Naturally, a specialist gets paid more than a general practitioner or a family doctor because he has spent a longer time in training for his specialty. So it's obvious to me that the government and President Kennedy's plan didn't work. A fifty-year-old policy should have been reevaluated and changed long ago.

The news media deserves much of the responsibility for the failure of the above plan too. The media was and is perfectly willing to report the various claims of government and to praise them instead of examining the issue for problems.

I have personal experience with another policy failure. During the seventies and eighties, my small group employed two doctors who had left the Soviet Union. Remember, the Soviet Union didn't allow their citizens to leave the country for many years. These two doctors had managed to escape allegedly with nothing to their name, not even their paperwork or their diplomas from universities. The state of California managed to allow these two doctors to get a medical license even without their diplomas. Can you imagine a US citizen's being able to get a license to practice medicine in any state without producing a diploma? We soon had to fire both of these doctors from the Soviet

Union. The first one, a man, was to help take care of our nighttime emergencies and urgent-care patients. He did do that but also was treating prostitutes in Hollywood over the phone, and they sometimes came to our small clinic and small hospital to see him and get narcotic prescriptions always at night when he was on duty and we were out of the office. With government so touchy about narcotics, this activity was unacceptable to our small family-practice-oriented group. We fired him and saw nothing more of him but did get a phone call from a detective in Chicago, asking if he was still in the area and if we knew where he was.

The second doctor from the Soviet Union we employed, a woman, who said she was a cardiologist, was fired after only a few months. The problem with her was that we were losing a lot of patients because of her forceful attitude toward the patients. She would order them to do this or that in no uncertain terms. That way might work in the Soviet Union but not in the United States. In addition, her personal hygiene was not up to our standard. She wore a long white lab coat that she seldom, if ever, washed when seeing patients. We also suspected that she seldom washed herself as her body odor overwhelmed anyone who walked into her office when she wasn't there and her lab coat was still in the room. Her methods of treating our cardiac patients were not standard in the United States either. We had many complaints from patients about the way she changed the treatments that they had been on for years and were working well.

After we fired the lady, she opened a solo practice a few miles from us. A few patients apparently followed her to her new practice. One of our regular and old patients came in to see me one day and told me that her mother was still seeing our ex-cardiologist. She told me then that she saw her mother's Medicare report of the cardiologist's billings and that she knew for certain that her mother had not had many of the tests and studies done that had been billed to Medicare. My patient then had encouraged her mother to change to another cardiologist. This was an incident that convinced me that the ethics of the former Soviet Union doctors was not up to our standards.

Let's touch on ethics a bit. We have lots of foreign-trained doctors in our area and on our hospital staff. Since they are all specialists, I often referred patients to them. Remember, they all have had their specialty training in the United States, so most of them are pretty competent in their field. The problem that bothered me was that often when I referred a patient for consultation in our local hospital, the consult was done, usually well, but when I saw my patient the next day, there would often be two or three more consults on the chart from other foreign-trained doctors of other specialties ordered by my original consultant. When I'm the attending physician, I'm the one who is in charge of any consults, and for the consultant to order further consults from his fellow countrymen without asking me is unethical. The reason this bothered me a lot is that this, of course, greatly increases the cost of the patient's medical care. In addition, I often had done or could do what the first consultant was asking the second and third consultants to do. This problem is another example of where our government's actions often have unintended consequences not necessarily good.

Another US policy I want to expose is about the Social Security Disability Program. About 1980, I was doing some evaluations for SS disability at SS's request. They would send me a form to report my findings after examining a patient they sent to me. One of the patients they sent to me to evaluate was the mother of one of my regular patients. My regular patient was a man who emigrated from Iran two or three years before this incident. His mother was in her early fifties and came to the United States about six months before I saw her. When the son brought her in to the examining room, he said he would interpret for her as she didn't speak any English.

I had a woman originally from Afghanistan working as a medical assistant at the time, so I asked her if she spoke the language (Persian) of the lady. She said of course she did, so I had the son wait in the waiting room while I took the history and examined his mother. The son was very unhappy about the change of interpreters. The mother said she had back pain. I examined her and found that she had no spasm and good motion of her back. I also did x-rays of her back and had a radiologist interpret them. The back x-rays were normal. The son was very disturbed that he couldn't stay in the room with his mother while I took her history and examined her. I later wrote up the report that I couldn't find any disabling problem with the lady. My problem with this incident is that a person only six months in this country, from a country that hates America and a religion that hates America and never paid into our SS system, is eligible to apply to SS for disability. Can anyone understand that policy of our federal government?

In the 1970s, the state of California, during the height of the malpractice insurance problem, required our medical office to post a sign prominently in the waiting room with instructions to the patient or others where and how to file a complaint against doctors and other medical personnel. Apparently, the state government's employees didn't have enough to do, or they wanted to hire more paper shufflers so their empire would be bigger. It seems to me that anyone not 100 percent satisfied with their visit to the doctor might be tempted to file a complaint but later not be inclined to because they had thought better of it or later understood more the reason for not being satisfied at first. At any rate, the requirement was mean and insulting to me as a physician trying to do my best for my patients. At the time, we were struggling to pay for our malpractice insurance, which had gone up in cost about 400 percent in one year. We were even without insurance for a year or so before our state medical association was able to form a good insurance company with more reasonable cost.

Several malpractice cases were filed against me over the many years I was in active medical practice in California. Most were about money. The plaintiffs were under the impression they could collect a large sum of money just because they wanted money. Some were angry at doctors in general. Some did collect a small sum of money to end the suit, or sometimes, it was easier and cheaper for the insurance company to pay a little than to spend months or years fighting it. A malpractice lawsuit usually takes about four years to run its course whether it's settled or goes before a jury.

Only one of the several suits filed against me went to a jury. The case was aimed more at my surgeon partner, but I was included because I was the assistant surgeon. The jury found in my favor. The plaintiff's attorney was very aggressive in his statements to the jury about my care of the patient, even distorting to the point of lies. So I was happy to be vindicated. I asked my able attorney if the plaintiff's attorney would have to be paid by the plaintiff or if he was working on a contingency basis and only got paid if he won the case and collected from us defendants or our insurance company. He told me that my insurance company would pay the plaintiff's attorney some money under some type of agreement. I was speechless and dumbfounded at that. This was an entirely unknown action as far as any known procedure in the lawsuit culture in my knowledge. This seems very much a conflict of interest if true, and I was convinced at the time of its veracity. Splitting fees in the medical profession has always been unethical, if not illegal. It surely must be unethical and likely illegal in the legal profession also. I, however, did nothing further to look into this issue because I was just happy to be cleared of the lawsuit and had planned to retire soon.

The malpractice suits filed against me were very upsetting emotionally to me. Knowing I had done nothing wrong and yet a suit was filed caused anger, denial, and depression. I found it very difficult to admit or talk about any lawsuit. This very likely affected my interpersonal relationships with my family, employees, patients, and colleagues. It's difficult to talk about to this day many years after retirement and the end of lawsuits.

I once had a patient admitted to our larger and well-equipped local hospital who claimed to be having headaches and other neurological problems, but I knew him to be a drug seeker and user. Nevertheless, he got admitted through the emergency room. I was, of course, obligated to evaluate him thoroughly. I couldn't find anything wrong with him after a very expensive workup with CT scans, consult with a neurologist, and consult with a neurosurgeon, a psychiatric consultant, and an internal medicine consultant. He was very vehement in his complaints and was demanding and getting a lot of narcotics during all the evaluations. He had no insurance, and after all the negative workup and the consultants telling me that he was faking his complaints to get drugs, the hospital told me he had to be discharged. It, of course, was my job to tell him the results of all the workup and that he had to be discharged from the hospital. He was quite angry and said he was going to sue me.

Later that same day, after he was discharged from the hospital, a lawyer called me about him. The lawyer said that the patient claimed I discharged him from the hospital with a fever of 104 degrees, that he went to another hospital who refused to admit him and then to the VA hospital who he said found a high fever too but didn't admit him either. The lawyer demanded information about the patient, or he was filing a malpractice suit against me. I became angry and told the lawyer that I had lots of consults, tests, and other information about the patient and that if he filed a suit against me, I would file a malicious prosecution suit against him. That was the end of that problem.

The US government should sponsor a major campaign against illegal drug use. It should include information about harm to the health of the drug user, the damage the drug dealers do to our society and the public, such as the associated violence, the expense of controlling the distribution, and the expense of treating the medical effects of the illegal drugs. Also, consider the cost to the taxpayer of controlling the smuggling across the border. Include the damage to other countries such as Mexico, Columbia, and others that have thousands of deaths each year due to the violence between gangs struggling to make more money and controlling the market. Emphasize that the illegal drug user is harming not only himself but also his family, friends, and society in general, especially his country.

This campaign should TV ads made by the professionals that can do such a good job, like the recent ads encouraging people to be nicer to one another. Also, perhaps sponsor lectures at high schools and universities to encourage people to get involved in convincing their family members and friends to avoid drug use. This campaign, if effective, would cut costs of border patrol, DEA, medical care, local policing, FBI, and prisons and cut drug-related violent deaths. It should improve trust in government because of less intrusiveness in the public's daily life. It would improve family life by taking away large reasons for family discord and strife between parents and children using drugs.

I admit there have been some campaigns before, but it needs to be done again and again. We see more campaigns against smoking than we do against drug use. The antismoking campaigns have been pretty successful over the years, so we should keep trying on the illegal drug issue. Our government has sponsored many other things less important with less impact than this would be.

There were lots of others, however. Plaintiff's attorneys

always demanded depositions, always under oath and with a court reporter. These depositions were a very intimidating way to harass the doctors and others, such as nurses or medical assistants, to push the doctor to agree to a financial settlement. A frequent tactic was to demand in the deposition that the doctor recount in detail all other lawsuits and complaints of me reported to the Medical Board of California.

I had no complaints with the Medical Board, but talking about previous malpractice suits was very distressing even when I had very little or no bad settlements or judgments. I eventually decided the lawyers would do whatever I let them, so I refused to answer any questions they asked about other malpractice lawsuits. That action made them angry, and they claimed they had the right to ask about any prior suits, and they would go to the judge and have him force me to answer. I told them to go ahead, that I didn't think the judge would let them continue to harass me in that way. They did go to the judge in more than one instance, and the judge only asked that I answer about other cases if they were related or about the same type of case. Of course, they were not, so I felt that I won that issue. All these demands from the plaintiff's attorneys were pure harassment attempts because all filed suits were public record anyway, and all they had to do was have a legal assistant do a computer search to get any and all information about any previous suits.

I also had my own defense attorney, assigned to me by the insurance company, ask and tell me in his initial interview with me that I must tell him about any previous lawsuits. Since I considered this part of the harassment too, I told more than once that I wasn't going to answer any questions or discuss any previous lawsuits. When they insisted that I answer, I told them that I was instructing them to take the position that I wasn't going to answer the questions about previous lawsuits and that if they couldn't defend that position for me, to withdraw from the case and have the insurance company assign another attorney. That ended the demands from my own attorneys and had none of them withdraw from my cases. Apparently, attorneys will do to you whatever you let them do and more.

CHAPTER 3

Various federal agencies have moved in the direction of controlling people's lives in the form of controlling their health by restricting what may be done for them. There are several examples of that.

Recently, there was lots of controversy about the prostate-specific antigen test (PSA). A federal commission came out with the recommendation that the test not be used. Many medical professionals disagree. The test is to detect prostate cancer early. Ostensibly, the commission says the test should not be used because it causes harm in some instances. First off, a test can't do harm. It's the use of the test result to plan and implement treatment that could possibly cause harm. The PSA has developed over quite a few years as a test for all men as they get past the age of fifty-five or so. Once the test is found to be elevated, it is checked and rechecked. Then other tests are done, which may be more specific in diagnosing or ruling out prostate cancer.

There is nothing wrong with doing a simple, inexpensive blood test as a screening for millions of men getting an annual physical exam. In fact, we would be negligent not to do so when such test is available because cancer of the prostate is very prevalent. I think that the federal commission was pressured by bureaucrats concerned about the cost of the PSA test done by millions on some type of government-paid health care or even on an HMO plan purely to save money at the expense of increasing the chance of men not detecting prostate cancer early enough to cure it or treat it properly. If there is any problem of overtreating cancer of the prostate as the commission implies, then the focus should be on the treatment issue, not the PSA test.

Further, this isn't the first time a commission or body of so-called experts has made recommendations that were obviously aimed at saving money at the expense of widespread increase in risk to health and even life. Pap smears have been a great method of detecting cancer of the cervix for over forty years now. But about twenty-some years ago, the American Cancer Society came out with a recommendation that the Pap smear not be done annually. Again, there was an outcry by practicing physicians that the test needed to be done annually as the cancer was a rapidly advancing type of cancer and was much better treated the sooner it was detected. Again, I think the panel of experts was pressured to make the less frequent test recommendation for purely financial reasons.

There was even a third incident of the same type. More recently, a commission of some "experts" said that women didn't need annual mammograms to detect breast cancer until past the age of fifty even though there are large numbers of women who are diagnosed and who die of breast cancer long before the age of fifty. Again, so obvious an attempt to save money for those insurance companies, HMOs, and various government-funded health care plans. Sorry, but saving money for some entity at the expense of life and health doesn't sit well with ethical, caring physicians. I always thought the science and art and the patient's well-being came before saving money, whether I was taught that in my formal training or not.

That brings up another issue, that of conflict of interest. Can't we see that HMOs especially have a conflict of interest in the way they manage paying for a patient's medical care? Note the news release about the founder and head of a large

HMO's retirement package of over a billion dollars a few years ago. He was ostensibly a doctor. How obscene since we all know the HMOs are known to withhold treatment or at least cut payments to doctors and others. There was very little outrage from the news media about it.

With all the problems of the government insurance companies and HMOs withholding treatment, I have no confidence that we won't have rationing of care when we have even more government control of medical care under the new health care plan. The same care for everyone at a much lower cost than now, without rationing care and restricting access, is wishful thinking and a myth.

Even our various government agencies have a conflict of interest in paying for medical care. They are charged with working within their budget and also paying the medical bills. Wouldn't it be better to have the patient and their doctor decide the limits of expense? Let me tell of some of the things done by third-party payers to our medical group.

We had a lot of poor people on Medi-Cal (Medicaid), the federal program for the poor to get the same care everyone else gets. We were required to bill electronically at one time far into the program. Our insurance billing employees would send a bill for our care of a patient electronically to the designated intermediary. We were supposed to be paid within three weeks of our billing. After the three weeks and not being paid, our billing clerk would call to ask why we hadn't been paid. The frequent answer was that they didn't receive the billing. Our clerk would send another bill exactly as before. Eventually, the intermediary would return the bill, saying that it was incorrect. Corrections, if any, were sent back by our clerks. Next, the payment might be sent after two or three times back and forth but at a reduced amount because the intermediary is saying that a less expensive service was provided instead of the one we billed for. They never ever said that we billed for a lesser service than we provided.

Further on this issue. After I retired, our state medical organizations filed suit against some of these intermediary payers and insurance companies and HMOs. These became class action cases with many doctors who had provided medical care for those companies' customers being part of the lawsuit. After several years of litigation, the companies were found by the courts to have underpaid the doctors according to their contracts. Three times I received a check for these underpayments. The checks were almost insulting in the amounts I received. I received only $75 to $250 in each instance. I had been cheated out of thousands of dollars in each instance. The lawyers got the lion's share of the settlements. What a cruel joke. To me, this shows dishonesty in not only our government but also in our businesses. What a shame on our country for allowing this. If it's done to our medical profession, it's likely done to many others too.

During the time I was taking care of Medicare and Medicaid patients, which was all the time I was practicing medicine in California with my partnership, we received from Medicare about 45 percent of our billings and from Medicaid about 28 percent. These payments were, of course, before all the hassle to get paid at all, the harassment, the denials, and the changes of the diagnostic code by their clerks to pay us a lower amount and the demands for frequent changes in such things as the way to bill them.

At least two times the billing procedures were changed. The result both times was a fiasco to get it done right both from our clerks' aspect and the intermediaries' payer. The changes were attempts to speed up and be more efficient in the processing of claims from physicians but ended up being much more difficult. Processing so many claims electronically sounds great, but most of the time, the changes were too soon for the attempt to work well.

Another example of changing to a new technology too

soon was when I was encouraged to renew my California medical license online. First off, I received no notice to renew it two or three months in advance as I was used to in the past. That alone is confusing, but I was diligent and caught the need to renew in time so I didn't have to jump through hoops to renew late when I would not be able to practice medicine until the renewal was done.

I logged on to the website, and it took me at least an hour and a half to complete the process even though there were instructions. I had to put in my information four times before the site accepted my information. If I had received the usual renewal through the mail, I could have filled out the renewal form, written the check, and mailed it in about five minutes. I'm sure many computer experts will laugh and say I need more computer skills. Well, that may be so, but I have listened to many computer-literate people describe the same type of problem and also read about many more.

Shouldn't these advances be easier instead of more difficult? Here's another thing: isn't it enough that I'm an expert in medicine so that I shouldn't have to be an expert in computers too? What if we require computer experts to also be experts in medicine? Silly, isn't it? I don't deny that computer use is very important. After all, our medical group has used computers since the early seventies. We bought a Basic Four with the promise that the computer would make our office much more efficient and less expensive. Not so. I asked the computer salesman if it would eliminate one of our many employees; he considered for a few minutes and said "Maybe one" of the twenty-some.

We were not able to do our work with even one less employee. The costs even went up considerably because now all the employees using the computer were now trained in the use of the computer and demanded higher pay because we had upgraded their skills. Our medical partnership had paid to train them the new skill after all. I think I'm not completely ignorant about computers since I've been working with them for so long. I've supervised my employees and certainly know what computers can and should be able to do but may not be able to do the operation on them myself. As a physician and a businessman, I should be able to hire any and all computer skills I need.

One of the reasons we bought our first computer was due to the state of California's beginning move to health maintenance organizations (HMOs). My managing partner, Dr. Tan, wanted to start an HMO, which would meet the state's plans to serve the Medicaid patients of the state, of which we had a large number. We consulted with the state's agent and eventually signed a contract with the state for the service to these Medicaid patients. We had many meetings with people on welfare and on the Medicaid program, spending a lot of money, but also getting quite a few patients. The plan paid us a flat rate for each patient we had each month. Problems started showing up soon after the program began. Often after we treated a patient, we would find out that the patient wasn't on the list of our patients that month. The state required us to treat the patient anyway if they weren't on the list just in case they were actually on the list but a mistake was made and they hadn't got the list correct. So we didn't get any money for that patient, and there was no recourse allowed. Many of these patients on Medicaid had very serious problems and required lots of medical care and hospitalizations, which we were obligated to pay for out of our monthly payment for each patient from the state.

One or more of the patients signed up in our HMO ended up in a hospital far from us with a drug overdose and ran up bills in the thousands of dollars, almost bankrupting us at the time. The final problem that came up that made me demand from my partner that we get out of the HMO business was when an agent of the state came to check on us to see if we were complying with the contract. After looking over our appointment book, he asked why one of the HMO-eligible patients didn't keep an appointment. Since we didn't know, our receptionist called the patient to ask why she didn't keep the appointment. The patient said that she didn't have a ride to our office. The state agent then told us that we would have to get a van to provide transportation for any of our HMO patients that needed a ride to our office or to a hospital or any other medical treatment facility that the patient needed. That requirement was never in the contract that we had with the state. Obviously, this would cost a lot of money to buy a van and to hire a full-time driver plus insurance. This is like changing the rules after the game is played and should have not been allowed but obviously was because it was done by a government and couldn't be corrected except by an expensive lawsuit.

Our profit margin was already very thin, if nonexistent. I told Dr. Tan that that was the last straw, and we ended our HMO attempt, losing a lot of money. Sure, I know someone will accuse me of being greedy, but look at it like this. Losing a lot of money on our HMO contracts would shortchange our other patients to make up the difference in money to run our office; that wouldn't be fair to them. No one can stay in business losing money all the time. That would be cost shifting, which we had already been doing and continued to do with our Medicare patients and our private-pay and insured patients.

Not all Medicaid patients were in that HMO, so we continued to care for them even though we barely broke even on their care. The HMO at the time seemed to draw the sickest patients and also the biggest users of medical care, like the drug addicts. Obviously, the state had convinced the welfare recipients that it was a good deal for them. The state obviously saw it as a good deal for them too by trying to shift the cost of those on the HMO roles to our private medical group. It worked for a couple of years until we caught on and ended our HMO. Many HMOs went on to make a lot of money. They likely had much smarter business sense than we did, or perhaps they learned by seeing our mistakes.

When I first got my California medical license, the annual cost was very low. Sometime in the 1980s, the cost was quadrupled. The reason was so the license fees would pay for investigators to investigate physicians. Don't get me wrong; I think there is a need for investigating and punishing doctors who do something wrong. But my one experience of an investigator convinced me they were approaching the issue wrong.

The investigator was checking on one of my nursing home patient's deaths and came on to me like I was a robbery suspect instead of a physician that had been caring for the patient in question. He gave me no chance to describe the problems the patient had, let alone what I had done for the patient. He just assumed if the very sick patient died, then I must have done something to cause the death. The investigators should be physicians or related health care professionals instead of policemen. The findings would be more realistic instead of looking clearly black-and-white. Medical issues are often not black-and-white.

About 1974, a very wealthy local family donated land in the middle of their housing developments to build a modern and major hospital for the community. There were already three smaller hospitals in our little valley and a major hospital only ten minutes away over the hill into the San Fernando Valley. All three small hospitals had room and plans to expand, but all eventually went out of business, likely due partly to the newspaper campaign about the supposed deficiencies of the smaller hospitals. The newspaper was owned by the same wealthy family that donated the land for the new hospital.

At the time, I couldn't disagree that an updated hospital was a good idea, so when asked to be on the board, I agreed to do so while the hospital was being built. After the new hospital was built, I was dropped from the board, about the time I was getting to know a lot about the way the board members were benefiting from the community hospital along with their friends. The board was then made up of 90 percent hospital managers and local businesspeople with a token doctor and the physician chief of staff that changed frequently. Notice that physicians who know the most about what patients need from a hospital were pushed aside in this instance and elsewhere in our area that I know of. This has come about from hospital administrators grabbing the power by dominating the board of governors of the hospitals. I think this is one of the reasons for the cost of medical care skyrocketing.

When I was in Idaho in the 1960s, the hospital board was happy to have the two doctors in town to come to the board meetings to talk about what was needed for the hospital to serve the community well. No more, now it's more to do with profit, even at so-called nonprofit hospitals. I have some reasons to conclude that opinion. My medical practice included a lot of industrial medicine, taking care of injuries on the job. The new larger hospital administrator hired a physician and opened a clinic near the industrial park to take the industrial patients' business in competition with many of the doctors on their staff. The administrator also opened other businesses in competition with the medical staff. One of them was a lab storefront to take tests from patients of nearby doctors' offices instead of the doctors' staff doing so. The hospital administrator also advertised widely for new doctors to come to the area even though there was no shortage of physicians in the area.

Sure, the administrator had every right to do those things, but it wasn't right for him to cause such dissension in the medical community. These problems caused divides in the medical community that was not good for the operation of the hospital. The hospital eventually went bankrupt, and the administrator lost his job. Much of the reason for the bankruptcy was the spending for the clinics and other businesses that were set up to take business that was traditionally done by doctors.

Another incident, even more damaging to the physicians in our area, was the CT scanner technology. When the CT scanner first came out, the state of California decreed that a "certificate of need" had to be obtained to get the new technology in a hospital. The state seemed to think that one CT scanner in LA County was enough. Of course, that was totally ridiculous as everyone knows now and we physicians knew then. Not being able to use the new technology when it was known about was totally unacceptable for us physicians as it would be negligent not to use it.

To get around the silly rule of the state health department, a group of about twenty of us local physicians put together enough money for the down payment of a CT scanner and rented space in the hospital for the scanner. The money received for the use of the scanner would pay for the loan to buy it. After upgrading to a better scanner at least twice, the loan was paid off after several years. The physicians that put up the initial money could then receive their money back and perhaps even make a profit on their investment. It was not to be. The hospital administrator discussed above gave the CT scanner group an ultimatum—either upgrade to a faster and much more expensive scanner, even though the scanner we had did essentially the same job, or he would not renew the lease on the room the scanner was in. That action essentially ended the CT scanner group's investment.

In the old days before insurance companies were put in charge of medical care and especially hospitalization, we doctors would often hospitalize a patient whose medical problem was unclear or uncontrolled. We would keep the patient in the hospital for several days if it looked helpful to do so. We used trained nurses, who in those days knew how to monitor and observe a patient to help us find out what was wrong and needed to be done. Also, we often did tests on the patient while the patient was still in the hospital, perhaps adding to the tests while the patient was being monitored. Sometimes we even tried new therapies or adjusted treatments while getting more information from the monitoring and observation to see what worked best for that patient. This kind of patient care and other similar caring actions by physicians and nurses is the reason the medical care in this country had the reputation of being the best in the world. Changing the process risks losing that good reputation.

Unfortunately for the patient, now the nurses are trained to keep records and untrained aides watch the patients occasionally. Thanks to the bureaucrats, the politicians, and the poorly trained health department's inspectors with their rules and requirements and their need to justify their jobs, the cost of hospitalization is too much for the taxpayer and insurance companies to bear, so a patient now can't stay in the hospital to be diagnosed or to recover enough from an illness or a surgery to manage well at home without a relative helping out even though the relative may not be qualified at all.

CHAPTER 4

Many changes have occurred in our society in the fifty years I've been a physician, many of them not good for our citizens.

Remember back in the 1960s, the ACLU filed a bunch of lawsuits against psychiatric hospitals and state governments to get patients discharged from the psychiatric hospitals. The reason was that the civil rights of the patients were being violated by keeping the patients in the hospitals against their will. I think the lawsuits sometimes had merit and sometimes not. After all, new drugs did help many patients to be much improved and able to live a more normal or traditional life. At any rate, the answer of the state governments and the psychiatric hospitals to the lawsuits was to discharge most of the patients and promise to provide outpatient care for the patients in the communities where they lived.

Unfortunately, the federal and state governments didn't and still don't provide the money or facilities in the communities for that outpatient care. This travesty is the main reason we have so many homeless for so many years. A large number of the homeless are either mentally ill or mentally deficient and unable to care for themselves properly. We as a compassionate society should be taking better care of these people either in well-managed outpatient clinics or, in some instances, in custodial care in psychiatric hospitals.

I recently toured some ex-psychiatric hospitals in Indiana where I had received some of my psychiatric training in medical school and found them in devastation with most of the buildings torn down and the rest in disrepair. I think there is still a place for many more of the mentally ill or mentally deficient to be cared for humanly in a custodial setting. It's not right to leave these ill people to exist on the street, living like animals because they are unable to cope properly for themselves.

There is another reason for more government intervention in the mentally ill or mentally deficient issue. That is the violence sometimes perpetrated by people with mental problems, usually not treated. We have seen atrocities in schools, malls, and workplaces where mentally ill people have killed several and sometimes many children and adults. Some of the blame for those incidents should be attributed to our government's failure to find and treat or control the mentally ill to protect other citizens. Many times, there have been multiple signs that a person is dangerous, but the signs were ignored by authorities. To be fair, the authorities also need legislation to be able do the right thing to protect the public from dangerous mentally ill people. Laws for involuntary commitment need to be revised.

Many people seem to go to an emergency room for their routine care, never realizing they are getting fragmented medical care by doing that. Going to their primary care physician is much more likely to provide the care that they expect. The emergency room is often busy, and nonemergencies will interfere with the efficiency of the real emergency and the emergency room will not provide the complete care that is needed by the nonemergency patient.

There seems no way to change the habits of our citizens in that regard. Perhaps the new health care law will eventually have to address that issue. The reason for not using an emergency room for general care is that the emergency service doesn't have an obligation to follow up on the patient's illness. Even going back to the emergency room initiated by the patient is not good because the physician on duty will be different. A private practice physician or a clinic will see the patient in follow-up, usually by the same doctor.

Our society has also seemed to move in the direction of wanting to see a specialist for their medical problems. Unfortunately, that often also is an inefficient way of getting top-quality medical care. For instance, I have often seen a patient decide that he needed a certain specialist for a symptom. The problem was not in that specialist's area of expertise. The patient didn't get the help expected and became disillusioned about our medical system, so he wants to change it to the government-run system. Instead, if that patient had gone to a generalist, discussed the problem, and then either been treated for the problem or referred to the appropriate specialist, he would likely have been more satisfied.

I believe the movement to consult a specialist first has been pushed by the news media and by the advertisements of lawyers to get patients to file class action lawsuits for questionable reasons. In addition, our news media constantly harps about the shortage of physicians, echoing our politicians and bureaucrats. I think that has a purpose, and that is to get socialized medicine in this country and hence control of the medical care by the government.

I believe that government policy is to intentionally cause the cost of medical care to go up so that the government can get more control. After all, it seems that government always wants to expand its control over more and more of society. The trend in this country is toward more socialism during my lifetime.

We've had a large influx of immigrants, most of whom came from countries with more socialistic governments, yet the immigrants fleeing a failed socialistic country for a perceived improvement by coming to the United States already want to change our system into what they left behind. Look at the Hispanics leaving their failed socialistic governments who mostly vote for the more socialistic Democratic Party in this country. This reason may be part of the movement to more government control of medicine in this country. We shouldn't give up something that's good about our country just to satisfy immigrants who don't yet understand the good and bad about their new country.

A few years ago, I was physician to a family who had come originally from communist Eastern Europe, escaping first to England, then to the United States. When the daughter had to have an appendectomy, the father lamented that he thought that it was bad that the United States didn't have a socialized medical system like England even though the family had only been in the United States for a year or so.

Organized medicine has responded poorly to the various attacks on our system of medical care. I think because there is often ambivalence from our medical leaders; after all, many of them are academics who are already government employees. We physicians have a sense that the professors know it all since we learned our basics from them. This sense is wrong. The physicians in private and active practice are likely more able than the professors.

For example, I often went to conferences and continuing medical education classes to learn new things and keep current in my field. Very often, the class was taught by a professor or instructor from a medical school, giving out advice about medical problems that I treated many times a day when the lecturer only treated rarely. After all, I saw upwards of forty patients a day while the lecturer was seeing perhaps five or six patients a day and teaching medical students the rest of the day. So who is the expert? I ask.

While we're on the topic of medical schools, I want

to criticize medical schools for their poor response to the shortage of physicians, if there is one. Our government spokesmen and our news media have been claiming there is a shortage of physicians for the fifty-some years I've been a doctor. Earlier I emphasized the importing of foreign-trained doctors to get specialty training and then keeping them here in the United States to alleviate the shortage. This began during the Kennedy administration and continues more than fifty years later.

It seems to me that medical schools should have increased their output of our own citizens to become doctors over that time. Surely, they could see the need. In these fifty years or so, the population of the United States has increased from about 160 million to over 300 million. In addition, there have been tremendous advances in the treatments and diagnosis and technology of medical care, requiring more physicians per capita of population. It's wrong to keep importing physicians from other countries. We should be training our own citizens to be doctors. Not to mention that we shouldn't be taking the brightest citizens from these other countries, which are poor and poorly developed, like the Philippines and India. When I did a tour of India, I had lunch at the home an Indian family. In the discussion, the man of the house indicated that he thought that there was a need for many more physicians in India. He was surprised that a large number of India's doctors have immigrated to the United States.

CHAPTER 5

There is great concern about the cost of medical care, especially in the speeches of our politicians and, of course, in the news media. I've observed many areas where the cost has been aggravated by the most vocal complainers, perhaps intentionally.

When I first went into private practice of medicine, it was illegal to advertise prescription drugs anywhere except to the doctors. Remember, the cost of medical care and medicine was much less then as I've described above, in the 1960s. Since then, our government has allowed the drug companies to advertise prescription drugs very extensively.

We all know that it costs a lot of money to advertise

on television. We are constantly bombarded with ads for one prescription drug or another if we have the television on. Think what that adds to the cost of that drug. If the drug is in widespread use, perhaps it doesn't add much to the cost to each prescription but still does add up. Many are ads for drugs used relatively infrequent that are very expensive. I am certain that those ads increase the costs for those drugs very significantly. The drug companies, of course, benefit hugely financially from those very expensive drugs. Just look at the tremendous profits reported by the multinational pharmaceutical companies. I don't begrudge a company for making a profit on their product, but when they do so in a way that I consider unethical, I feel justified in criticizing the action. Our federal and state governments seem quite happy with the high costs and profits; after all, the governments benefit by more tax money that way.

There is also the issue of whether it's right to interfere with the doctors' and patients' interactions and decisions. The advertising of prescription drugs does that in a big way. I have had many, many times when a patient has come to me asking to be prescribed a drug they've seen advertised on TV. Very often, those drugs were either inappropriate or only a more expensive drug that does the same thing as the drug the patient has already been taking. After all, if the newer or more expensive advertised drug was more helpful or indicated for the patient, I would have already advised using it from my knowledge of what the patient needed. Many times, the advertised drug's benefits are grossly exaggerated, distorting the patient's perception of the need or benefit they might receive. These problems with the drug advertising convince me that prescription drugs should not be advertised to the general public as the public does not have the ability to judge the issues. If we as a society are dissatisfied with the cost of drugs and medical care, then this issue should be addressed to help lower the cost of both drugs and medical care.

When I was an army physician, it was often impressed on us physicians that we should be aware of the cost of the drugs we prescribed as the army didn't want to go over the budget for that item. The army generally bought the cheapest generic drugs available. These drugs sometimes had to be used in double dose to do the job expected of them. As an example, I used a broad-spectrum antibiotic for sinus infections (tetracycline), which was a generic made in Italy. I had to use double the recommended dose to get the desired effect on the disease. One year in the spring, the pharmacist came to our ENT clinic and told us that he had a budget surplus and could get us some brand-name antibiotics for a time. We were able to get a brand-name tetracycline that was effective at the recommended dose.

Another issue related to the army has to do with the expiration dates on prescription drugs. The *Wall Street Journal* published an article on March 28, 2000, by Laurie P. Cohen that reported a study by the US military. The study was done because the military was spending a lot of money on drugs that often had to be discarded at a stated expiration date and fresh drugs bought. The study was to find out if the drugs were still effective after the expiration date and how long they were effective. The testing was done by the Food and Drug Administration and included over one hundred drugs. About 90 percent of the drugs tested were safe and effective for many years past their stated expiration dates, some as much as fifteen years past it. This brings up the question if the drug companies are exaggerating the short shelf lives of drugs for financial reasons only.

Over the years since, I haven't seen any discussion of this issue by any government agency, the pharmaceutical industry, or the various news media. Why not? Don't the general public deserve to know that they may be being overcharged for their drugs by labeling of expiration dates that are not calculated on scientific data and reasoning?

There are widespread consequences of this deception, such as poor countries that need drugs for their people reject donated drugs if they are within a year of their expiration dates on the labels because of the urging of the World Health Organization. There are many others. Much good could be done if the pharmaceutical companies and the regulatory agencies would do a better job of determining when a drug actually loses enough potency or develops toxicity to justify an expiration date.

Another area of wasted money in our medical care system is in the area of surveyors and inspectors in the health departments of various governments. I think that an example in my personal experience will best show that. I was the medical director of a ninety-nine-bed nursing facility for at least twenty-five years. Numerous times, a health department inspector, or often named a surveyor, would come to the facility and make evaluations and recommendations. It was often obvious that many of those recommendations were to show his power and to justify his job. Most of the recommendations were not actually recommendations but demands that the facility was obligated to do. One of the recurring demands was to advise that a physical therapist and an occupational therapist come into the facility and evaluate whether each and every patient was getting all the physical and occupational therapy that they needed or could use. These demands had to be done even when I or other doctors had already taken care of those needs.

Invariably, the physical and occupational therapists would put on the patients' charts that this or that should be done. Many times, these things being advised were not needed and even inappropriate for patients in very compromised health and situations. However, it was very difficult for the physicians to counter the recommendations of these consultants because the health department's employees are considered the final authority, and physicians risk investigation and loss of their medical license if they don't follow recommendations of consultants. Observe that the physical and occupational therapists have much less training in medicine than the physicians. Not to mention that the health department inspectors or surveyors may have no medical training at all and sometimes only rudimentary advanced education.

I was chairman of the audit committee for several years for our major local hospital. The purpose supposedly was to identify problems within the hospital environment and improve them. It was actually a committee that put together studies that were totally worthless for getting any improvements to patient care. These audits were required by the Hospital Accreditation Commission, who came to the hospital every year to survey and give the hospital its accreditation for participation in the Medicare program. After the several years of monthly meetings, I concluded that the committee was just a make-work facade to look good on paper but of no real value. I would have been of much more use seeing patients during those many hours in the meetings. If we're going to control the cost of medical care, these types of problems must be resolved too.

There have been lots of exposures of fraud in the Medicare and Medicaid programs reported in the news media. There has been fraud by doctors, hospitals, and many other providers. One of the ones widely reported was the supplying of motorized wheelchairs to disabled people. The electric chairs only cost about $1,000. But it was reported that some suppliers were billing Medicare ten or twenty times that amount. Granted Medicare always pays less than they are billed, but that was ridiculous and clearly fraudulent, and apparently, Medicare paid some exorbitant claims anyway before someone noticed the fraud, giving us a hint of the quality of the Medicare employees making the payments.

The doctors committing fraud usually billed Medicare for procedures they didn't do, sometimes paying "patients" a portion to let them claim the procedures were done. It's easy to see why some doctors would stoop to fraud because of the way Medicare and Medicaid always cut legitimate billings drastically and stalled about paying on time. But there is no amount of money worth losing your freedom.

I have no doubt there is lots of fraud, including citizens who aren't really disabled but are able to claim and get Social Security disability payments by faking or exaggerating their symptoms and problems. If they are turned down on their first attempt, all they have to do is get a lawyer to file appeal after appeal until they get a sympathetic clerk in the disability claims office to approve the claim. I've seen it happen.

I think our government has done a poor job of paying legitimate claims properly and then missing a lot of fraudulent claims. The government needs to improve its payment procedures if we're going to continue to have a first-rate medical care system in this country paid for largely by government programs. It seems that we do need the government to be a watchdog in this instance. We also need to have a watchdog system for the HMOs and other insurance schemes that have cheated patients and doctors in a big way with the complicity of the government.

Why has our society allowed the destruction of our

excellent private medical care system? Money is the basic reason. At the same time, we seem to have a distorted sense of priorities. For instance, one of the most blatant distortions of priorities is the acceptance of pay in advance and through the nose for entertainment but expecting to pay little and months or even years later for medical care and, even then, wanting someone else, like insurance or government, to pay. We have to pay for TV cable or TV satellite service in advance. We pay $12 or so to go to a movie for a two-hour show where there are hundreds of patrons in the same room. Also, we pay $100 for a play that may have thousands in the same room. All paid in advance. Entertainment often seems to take priorities over shelter and food sustenance. I think this is mostly an American attitude.

In this country, we seem to expect and often demand a discount for everything we buy, including services. Maybe this is the reason we also want a discount on our medical and health care and then accept nurse practitioners and physicians' assistants at a lower level of medical care than doctors are trained to provide.

There has been a movement, with pressure, to have clinicians follow protocols for many diseases. The plan seems to be for a panel to decide which therapies have worked best for the ones on the panel and make that the protocol for that disease. After forty-five years of practicing medicine and another twelve of watching the way medical practice is going, I can attest that diseases and medical care are seldom standard. Sure, immunizations can be mostly standardized but not most cancers, pneumonias, injuries, infections, or emotional problems and many other things too numerous to list. It's wishful thinking on the part of the professors and others that think they are better able to tell what's best for the masses.

Our federal government agencies and some state agencies as well have caused a great deal of turmoil in the medical profession by their efforts to control narcotic use. They have pressured and prosecuted doctors and pharmacies not to prescribe narcotics. Unfortunately, many patients have trouble getting pain relief because of their doctor's reluctance to come under scrutiny for his prescribing habits. Of course, drug abusers should be controlled and punished, including doctors who prescribe narcotics without good reason.

My observation is that the federal government has been overzealous in their pressuring and prosecutions. A few years ago, the California legislature mandated that all California-licensed physicians take a continuing medical education course on the appropriate use of narcotics and pain relief. Ignoring that those clinicians prescribing narcotics for their patients already knew all that and many physicians didn't even use narcotics for their patients, often because of their specialty, such as radiologists. What a waste of time and expense and, of course, an interference in a legitimate profession.

I often encounter claims that computers and other electronic technologies in a doctor's office cut the cost of medical care. Our federal government is now claiming that the digitization of all medical records will lower the cost of care. I don't believe it. Consider the purchase cost, installation, training, maintenance, frequent updating, replacements, and retraining. The computer industry's tendencies for extremely frequent updates, breakdowns, replacement requirements, retraining when they update, and very quickly stopping to support recent technology will prevent any financial advantages. In addition, I can't believe that these records put in a national database will be secret and secure. We all know that all sorts of governments will demand access so they can produce all kinds of data that will purport to benefit us all. We've done well without all that data for years and years. Nowadays it's about documentation. It used to be about the patient. If the doctor is fooling with the computer, he's not giving his full attention to the patient and his problems.

A great deal of money claimed as costs for medical care don't actually go to medical personnel. I'm referring to administrators, insurance company profits and administrative costs, social workers, home health aides who actually do housework, drivers of transport vans, nutrition advisers, and many others. These costs have been added to the calculated costs of medical care, seemingly to jack up the perceived costs so our citizens will be outraged at the increasing costs out of line with inflation.

It looks to me like the tactic worked. Consider the new laws passed in the last two or three years that are untested but appear to be only more regulation and coercion from the bureaucrats that can only increase the cost of medical care in the long run. Those new laws and regulations can only decrease access to medical care. I think we will soon see even more rationing of medical care.

Some people tell me that they pay $2,000 to $3,000 a month for medical insurance for the family. I can't imagine a healthy family, which most families are, paying nearly that much if they paid cash and bought catastrophic insurance instead with a large deductible insurance. Much of these costs go to insurance company profits.

Way back in the nineties, the federal government prohibited Medicare balance billing by doctors. In other words, doctors could not collect or accept from Medicare patients more than Medicare approved for the service provided. If a doctor who accepted Medicare treated a senior who opted out of Medicare, he could only charge the patient the approved Medicare rate or he could go to jail.

I bring this up because Medicare payment rates are so low that they barely pay for a doctor's costs to provide care. This, of course, has been going on for many years. In my many years of practice, I wouldn't have been able to care for Medicare and Medicaid patients if I didn't also have patients paying cash, other insurance, industrial injuries, employment exams, and several other sources of income. This has been called cost shifting. As you can imagine, many of these other sources of income eventually got tired of this cost shifting and put an end to it. Hence, HMOs and other watchdogs were eventually authorized and protected by Congress to follow the lead of Medicare and Medicaid to cut their payments to doctors and hospitals to levels that often didn't even equal the costs of providing care.

No individual or corporation can stay in business when their incomes are consistently below what it costs them to run their business. That caused large numbers of hospitals to have financial problems, many going bankrupt and many making changes in the way they did business. Both for-profit and not-for-profit hospital changes sometimes involved limiting services, expanding outpatient services that might be more profitable, rationing care, which involved sending patients home earlier, and a few others. Not surprisingly, many of those changes lowered the quality of their patients' care. In addition, some of those hospital changes invaded traditional physicians' areas of responsibility. For example, a local hospital rented an office in an industrial area and hired a physician to staff it in competition to me and other physicians who were treating industrial-injury patients. Of course, this made it more difficult to cost shift and make a profit because industrial-injury patients usually were more profitable than a Medicare or a Medicaid patient.

I want to touch on the issue of gifts to doctors by vendors such as drug companies' detail personnel. For many years, physicians would receive sample drugs and other promotional items such as ball-point pens with the company name and occasionally more valuable items such as a T-shirt or a little toy with their company name. The drug samples, of course, were important to patients as the doctor could give the patient a sample to get started, see if the drug was tolerated or helpful and even cut the cost to the poor patients having difficulty paying for the drug. Sometimes a drug company or equipment company would pay a physician's way to a conference promoting their product, but also, the conference would be educational for the doctor. Congress, quite a few years ago, passed a law making it illegal for physicians to receive any gifts over a dollar or two in value. The ostensible reason for the law was that this was bribing the physician to use the drug or equipment. To me, this type of control was very insulting as an ethical person would not prescribe or use a product for their patients if it wasn't needed or appropriate. I think it even was insulting to the whole profession of physicians. I consider the vast majority of doctors in this country to be ethical and act primarily in their patients' best interest.

Many times patients expect more than a physician can do. This leads to complaints and lawsuits. I think a lot of over expectations come from movies, news stories, and novels. For example, I once had a patient who had some vague symptoms. When I evaluated him, I found he had Hodgkin's disease, a treatable problem. I referred him to an oncologist for treatment. When I saw him in the hospital the next morning, he was irate at the oncologist and me but couldn't express what we had done wrong.

The constant attacks on medicine that I have seen

have damaged the quality of medical care in this country and definitely damaged my pride and satisfaction in the excellence of my profession and my own personal work and career. This destruction of a very good system has been just so the socialists can get control of a large segment of our economy. If that's the system our citizens want, then they should now live with it and stop complaining. If it turns out that our citizens don't like the system, then blame the politicians that rendered it and not the physicians.

CHAPTER 6

Here is an example of the differences between a foreign country's medical care and our American medical care. It is my own experience.

Sometime in January 2002, my next-door neighbor and friend, Don, asked me if I wanted to go on the sailboat race from Newport, California, to Ensenada, Mexico, in April. I gave an enthusiastic yes. I had been on a few races to Catalina from Long Beach with Don in 2000. However, he had stopped racing in 2001. I'm not much help on a sailboat except to pull a rope now and then under the direction of other crew members, but I enjoyed the trips with Don and other crew members.

Don was eighty-two years old and slowing down a bit,

and with enough crew that knew how to sail, I was happy to go along as a passenger or for my medical ability. Two weeks before the Newport-to-Ensenada race, Don decided to participate in the race from Long Beach to Catalina and back which we did with two other crew members, Bill and Alan. We did rather poorly but at least knew a few things that we needed to correct and add for the Ensenada race. I had helped Don with a few repairs on his boat previously, which included repacking the propeller shaft using my scuba gear and ability and a few other minor repairs and adjustments to the boat. His boat was a thirty-seven-foot wooden-hulled boat built forty to fifty years ago named *Blue Bell*.

The evening before the race was to start, I drove down with Don and loaded the boat with our provisions and personal gear. I found Don to be a little bit forgetful at that time. More than once, he said he couldn't remember if he put his shoes in or this item or that item, but generally, he drove down well and functioned normally otherwise. Don and I stayed aboard the *Blue Bell* the night before the race. I slept well as usual aboard a gently rocking craft. However, Don stated that he slept very poorly that night.

The morning of the race, we were joined by crew members Alan, Bill, and Roy, all experienced sailors with Don. We had a long motoring run from San Pedro to Newport for the start of the race. There were several hundred boats in the race, somewhere between four hundred and five hundred, I'm told, with about twenty-five in our class. Our class was a cruising class, which would include the ability to run with a motor during certain parts of the race if necessary.

The race started well. We crossed the start line fairly quickly at one thirty in the afternoon. There were some classes ahead of us and some classes behind us with different start times. The wind was strong, and the crew quickly put up sails and constantly trimmed them to get the maximum speed in the proper direction. We had a mainsail up, a Genoa sail, and a staysail. We sailed all afternoon and all night with moderately heavy seas and a strong wind. At some point during the night, we had to reef the mainsail to help control the boat. Don, Roy, Alan, and Bill managed the helm at different times during the afternoon and night. During the night, almost no one got any sleep because of the rough seas. Don, however, was in his bunk part of the night. I also lay in a bunk but could not sleep. I was wedged in from behind a brace to keep from being thrown out when we hit heavy swells. During the night, Don was up out of his bunk with vomiting and diarrhea, which might have contributed to what happened later or might have been the beginning of his problem.

At daylight, we were still doing well, going five to seven knots as we approached Ensenada. However, as we came inside the islands with Ensenada coming into view, the wind died down perhaps five miles short of the finish line. We saw a few sails ahead of us and a large number of sails behind us. We had passed up a few of the running lights within sight of us during the night. The wind died, so we proceeded at a relatively slow rate with the crew working hard to catch every puff of wind by various adjustments to the sails and trimming frequently. As we got closer to the finish line, numerous boats were becalmed, but we slowly drifted toward the finish line, and just before we got there, we were able to catch a slight breeze and sailed across the line nicely. While the sailing crew took down the sails, Don started the motor to go to a mooring, but then we began to see the first of the problems when Don, a longtime sailor, went around a red buoy on the wrong side. We then motored into the harbor and anchored, with Don at the helm.

We arrived at Ensenada at approximately 8:30 a.m. Shortly after anchoring, Roy hailed a shore boat and went ashore to take a shower and get cleaned up. The rest of us started putting away sailing gear and had some breakfast. At that time, we began to notice that Don was having trouble with some coordination and memory as he asked us more than once about breakfast, and he had difficulty moving around the boat and doing such things as opening a box of cereal. We talked it over among the crew and decided it was a very fatiguing night for Don, with him being sick during the night and not sleeping for at least two nights. He was resistant to the idea that he was not normal, but we eventually convinced him to lie down and rest for several hours. Roy and I then went ashore to turn in the engine log, and I stopped by a pharmacy to buy some glucosamine that Don had forgotten to bring with him, which he took for his joint pains.

When I got back on board about 2:00 p.m., Don was awake and up. It seemed to me that Don was no better. He was forgetful, disoriented, and seemed to have difficulty with his vision then. He also became verbally abusive and angry when I mentioned his symptoms, denying that there was anything wrong. I tried to lie down and rest so I wouldn't precipitate angry outbursts from Don but couldn't because I was worried about him. I got up and discussed the situation with Bill and Alan. Roy was still ashore. It seemed to me that Don had had a stroke. The visual problems, coordination difficulties, and even the anger and verbal abusiveness are often symptoms of strokes. He argued vehemently that he was all right and wouldn't go ashore with me to see a doctor. He finally agreed after much discussion that I would go ashore and call his wife, Dottie, to see what she had to say about the symptoms.

I went ashore to make the call, but finding a telephone that I could call through to California was difficult. Our cell phones would not work in Mexico. I eventually found a pharmacy some distance from the harbor that had long-distance service. After several attempts, I got through to Dottie about 8:00 p.m. I told her the problem. She said to tell Don to do whatever I told him to do. Bill had gone to the race committee at the Bahia Hotel requesting assistance and was told to go to the San Jose Hospital there in Ensenada for help. He had also determined at the time that there was no ambulance or paramedics to help if we wanted to remove Don on a litter. I told Dottie of this plan if we could get Don to get off the boat for that. I returned to the boat where Don was still very resistant to getting off the boat, but he finally agreed to get off the boat and talk to Dottie on the phone. Of course, I also planned to take him to the hospital to get checked while we were ashore.

The logistics of getting a man who had lost his

coordination off a sailboat onto a shore boat and then onto the dock was quite difficult physically, even after I had managed to convince Don that it was necessary. I think he finally began to realize that there was a problem when he encountered the problems getting ashore. The people operating the shore boat service were very helpful in getting Don ashore and into the taxi. He didn't argue as much getting into a taxi to get to the pharmacy with the long-distance telephone.

By the time we got all the convincing and transporting done, the pharmacy with the long-distance phone was closed for the night. Other pay phones, including the one at the race committee headquarters at the Bahia Hotel, would not or could not provide long-distance service to the United States.

We told the taxi driver we wanted to go to the San Jose Hospital, but he didn't seem to know where it was. He stopped at a phone booth and asked someone but still didn't know where to take us. He did eventually take us to another pharmacy that was open and had long-distance service to the United States. The pharmacy didn't know where the San Jose Hospital was either. By then, we began to get a bad feeling.

While we were waiting for the taxi driver to try to find

the San Jose Hospital, we got Don into the phone booth by half carrying him. He talked to Dottie, who told him to do whatever I told him to do. He finally became compliant and no longer belligerent. I also talked to Dottie, who had tried to call the San Jose Hospital, but the phone operator didn't know of any San Jose Hospital in Ensenada but did find a San Jose Clinic. When Dottie tried to talk to the clinic, the nurse didn't speak English and the doctor was not available. Dottie also had tried to set up an air ambulance to fly to Ensenada to pick up Don and fly him to the Los Angeles area for medical care.

However, at the pharmacy, in the meantime, I had found out from the pharmacist that the airport in Ensenada was not open to the public and was only open to the Mexican Army. Therefore, the air ambulance wasn't going to work unless we could get Don to the Tijuana Airport. We had long discussions about whether we should try to get to Tijuana either by taxi or take the boat and motor to Tijuana, which, being one hundred miles away, would take several hours and would be stressful to Don. The discussion also included that if we could get him to a hospital and evaluated, perhaps the hospital could help us get an air ambulance into the Ensenada Airport because of an emergency.

During the conversation with Dottie on the phone at

the second pharmacy we found, she said she had also talked by phone to the US Consulate in San Diego and that the personnel there could possibly help us get across the border expeditiously. At this point, Don had difficulty talking on the phone, he had difficulty managing the transferring of the phone from one hand to the other, and he had difficulty walking and seeing. As you can see, all of us were desperately trying to get help for a seriously ill man. After Dottie told Don to "please do whatever Clyde suggests," he became cooperative. Dottie told me to do whatever it takes to get care for Don.

We returned to the taxi. The driver thought he now knew how to get to the San Jose Hospital, which turned out to be the San Jose Clinic with no doctor and possibly closed. We directed him to take us to any hospital that he knew that would take emergencies, which he proceeded to do. When we got to the hospital, the name of which I cannot recall, the main entrance was quite nice and seemed to be fairly new. The automatic sliding door did not open, and we had to pull them apart manually at the direction of the taxi driver.

Inside the reception area was a receptionist / phone operator who did not understand English, but again, the taxi driver was able to help by interpreting for us. The doctor came out of the emergency department to meet us. He was a young man who appeared to be about fifteen years old to me, but he did speak English and was very nice and helpful. There was no wheelchair to get Don from the taxi to the emergency room, so we again half carried him to an examining table. I told the doctor that I was a doctor and gave him the history and symptoms that I had observed. He checked Don's blood pressure and did a brief neurological exam, finding his blood pressure elevated to 160/100. He gave Don some sublingual captopril to bring the blood pressure down. I asked the doctor if he had a CT or MRI scanner available. He said, "I wish I did, that's why I want to go to the United States to work." With this information, Bill and I decided that we should get Don back to the United States as fast as possible and not continue to try to get care for him in Mexico as it was taking a long time and not likely to be successful in getting a good outcome. We decided to call Dottie to tell her the plan.

We went to the hospital telephone operator, but none of us had enough Spanish ability to tell her what we wanted, but the taxi driver came to our rescue again to interpret. He was waiting for us at the door. He told the telephone operator that we wanted to call California. She informed us that they had no method of getting through to California from their switchboard. This was not only surprising but also depressing as this was a modern-appearing hospital in a relatively popular resort city. The taxi driver said, "That's no problem, let's use the pay phone in the lobby and have the operator reverse the charges." We went to the pay phone, but no operator would come onto the line. Our helpful driver said, "Let's try another phone." We went down the street, tried two more pay phones, but still could get no operator.

It had occurred to us to get Don transferred to the United States by ambulance, but in our discussions with one of the pharmacists earlier, we had been informed that that was very unlikely. I asked the taxi driver if it was possible for us to get to Tijuana or San Diego by taxi. He said yes, he would take us to San Diego for $200. I thought this was our best option as my son Lloyd lived in San Diego, and if I could get a hold of him, we could get him to meet us near the border and take us all the way back to a hospital near home in a shorter time than it was taking to get good care in Mexico. I told the taxi driver that I would give him $300 to take us to San Diego, but I needed to go back to the boat to get my gear and my cell phone so I could get Lloyd on the phone to arrange a meeting place on the freeway in San Diego.

I then told the doctor in the emergency room my plan to take Don to San Diego by taxi, and he approved of the plan. We got Don back into the taxi and paid the bill for the emergency room visit. It turned out to be, 400 Mexican pesos, which was about $45. The taxi driver took us all back to the dock where Bill and I went back to the boat, and I picked up my gear and cell phone. I told Roy the plan as he was on board again. We went to the Bahia Hotel, and with the help of a race committee staffer and the hotel telephone operator, we were able to call Dottie and Lloyd and finalize the plan. By then, it was after midnight, and Lloyd would meet the taxi near the border in San Diego after we crossed the border, and I could use my cell phone to arrange the place to meet. The taxi driver could then return to Ensenada. At this point, our very helpful taxi driver said that he was unable to cross the border as he did not have the proper card but that another driver did have the card to cross the border. The new driver did not speak much English but apparently received adequate instructions from the original driver as things went well. The driver transfer was done. I gave the original driver a big tip in appreciation for his great help. I wish the American race committee had been as helpful as this driver.

At about 1:00 a.m., Don and I finally got started back

toward San Diego in the taxi. This transfer went well. The line at the border was only about a fifteen-minute wait. Once we got across the border, my cell phone worked within a mile or so. I found out at this point that the number I had programmed in my cell phone for my son was his home number and not his cell phone. He had already left home to meet us, so he was on the road. I also found out that the cell phone number he had for me was not my new cell phone number. This left us with no direct way to talk and meet. I called home to talk to Daniele to get Lloyd's cell number. The line was busy. I called our second line, which she answered. She was on the other line with Lloyd, so we got each other's number to be able to communicate.

He was on the freeway behind us. We made an off ramp and told Lloyd where we were and shortly were able to meet and transfer the gear and Don to his car. Lloyd, being fluent in Spanish, was able to tell the taxi driver how to get back to the border expeditiously. I paid the taxi driver the promised $300 and a big tip in appreciation. I am glad I had taken a lot of cash on the trip as I couldn't have done all that was necessary at this point with checks or credit cards. We were then on our way back north to Don's family and doctor.

By the way, almost all the people we asked for help

in Mexico were as helpful as they could be under the circumstances, with a few exceptions. The biggest exception was the Californians who were the race committee who told us to go to the San Jose Hospital when there was only a clinic, which was not prepared to see our kind of problem and did not have an English speaker on duty. Also, the Bahia Hotel didn't let us use a long-distance phone when we first tried, and when we did finally get the race committee people to get us permission to use the phone, it was at the desk where the receptionist told me it would cost $1.25 per minute and very noisy next to all the sailors partying. I didn't care about the cost when it was an urgent matter. I could barely hear Dottie and Lloyd on the phone.

The transfer in Lloyd's car from San Diego to Holy Cross Hospital in Granada Hills went almost without incident. Don slept most of the way, but when he woke up, he was confused, wondering what all the cars were doing around us and why we were driving him around all over the place. Also, he kept asking why Alan didn't drive him in his car even though we explained more than once to him that Alan's car was not in Ensenada but in San Pedro. As we came through the center of Los Angeles, Don began to have a headache over his right temporal area. Around this time, I called Dottie and asked her to meet us at Holy Cross

Hospital at 5:00 a.m. where we finally obtained modern medical assistance.

Don was hospitalized, and tests were started immediately. I had Lloyd take me home where I went to bed for some sleep as I had not slept for two nights. Don did have a stroke and spent three weeks in the hospital for treatment and rehabilitation. He never recovered completely and died about two years later. We spread his ashes in the Pacific Ocean.

We later found out that we had won our class in the race (Cruz Spin B), 125 miles in 19.9769 hours, a fine ending for Don's career as an engineer and sailor. Bill and Alan sailed the *Blue Bell* back to San Pedro the next day. Roy brought the beautiful trophy home by car.

Please see the photos.

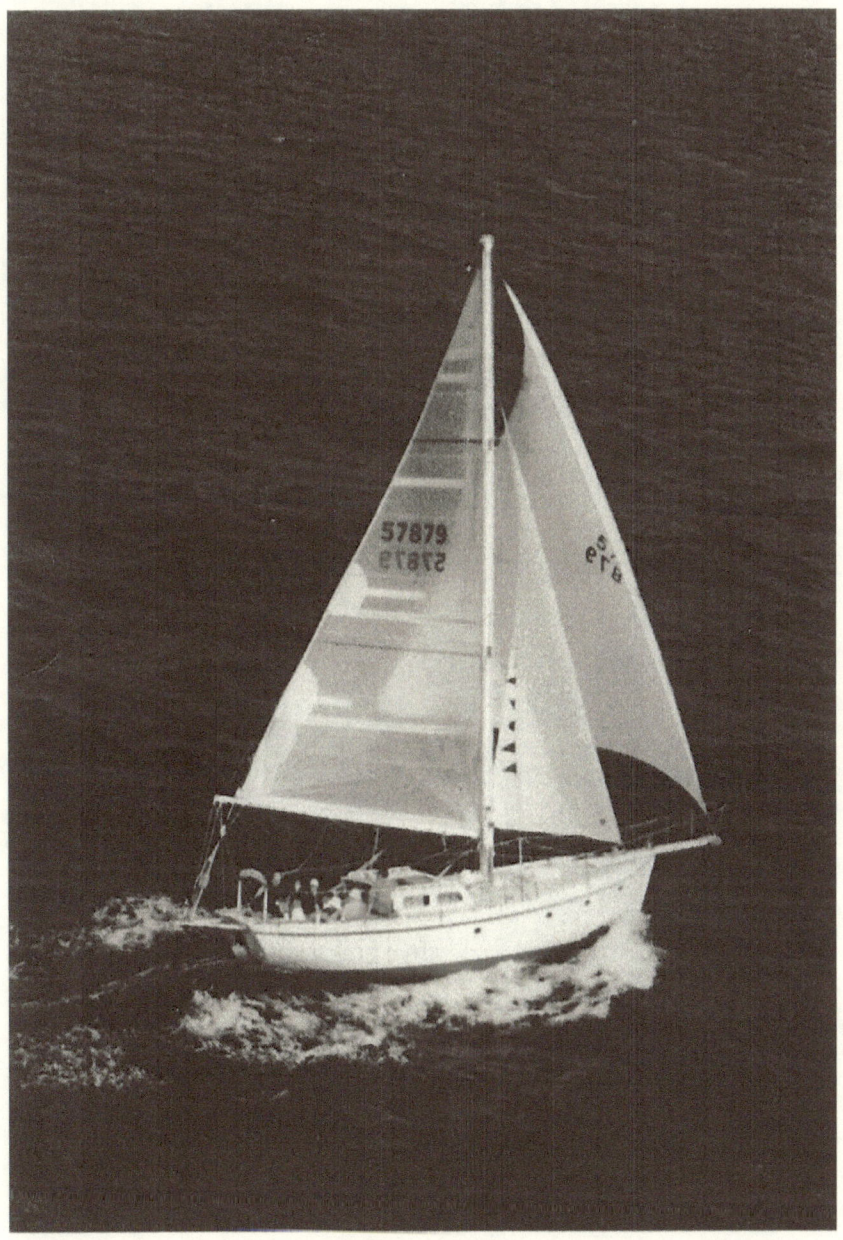

Blue Bell

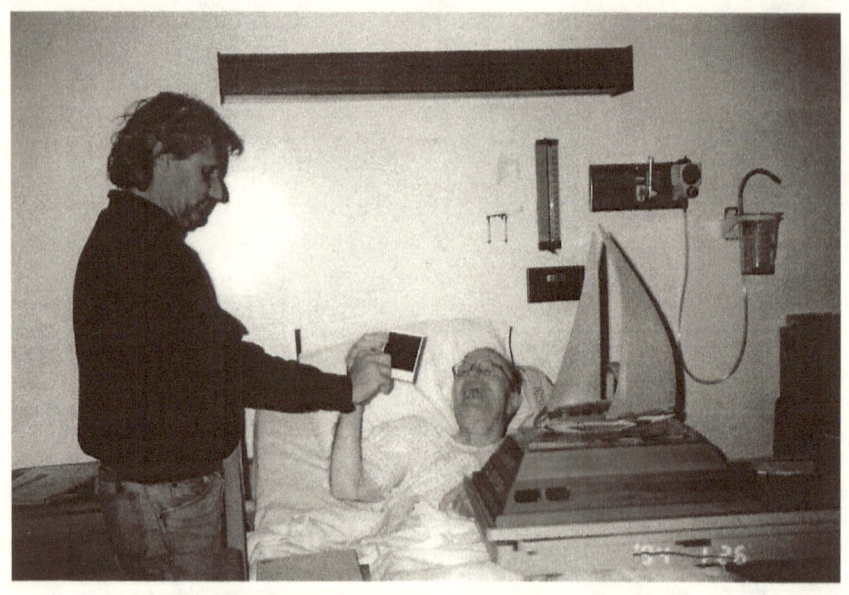

Don and Allan with trophy

PART 2

CHAPTER I

This essay is a parody that I wrote some time ago as an illustration of the controls on and coming onto the medical profession that I considered very intrusive and harmful.

The outlandish escalating cost to fans of sporting events to attend games and events or even listen to or watch events on television has precipitated the following proposal.

The United States government will form a new cabinet-level Department of Sporting Events. The department will consist of a department head or secretary of sports and forty-seven undersecretaries. A new undersecretary may be added each time a new sport is added to the department's responsibility. Each undersecretary will supervise up to forty thousand departmental employees the first year. If more employees are needed, the undersecretary may not add more than the prior year's total staff each year. In other words, each underdepartment may only double each year.

The new Department of Sporting Events' (DOSE) responsibilities will be to supervise all sports in the United States. All players, coaches, referees, announcers, grounds men, flaggers, clerical workers, scorekeepers, and anyone else involved in any sports will be paid by the department as employees. In implementing its new procedures, the new department (subsequently referred to as DOSE) may not lower the pay scales of any of its supervisees (herein further referred to as the department's other personnel easily supervised or [DOPES]).

The DOPES's current salaries are guaranteed for the first three days to be the going rate. However, if DOSE finds the price of the salaries too high to pay, any of the staff of DOSE with a rating of GS-3 or higher may order the pay of any DOPES cut to what the staff member thinks is fair pay. Otherwise, DOSE will pay 100 percent of the DOPES's salary for the first three days, then will pay 10 percent less each three-day period after. The salaries will be reevaluated each three and a half days for fairness by a committee of forty of each subdepartment of DOSE.

An appeal process will be available to ensure fairness

for the DOPES. An appeal written in the DOPES's own handwriting must be submitted to each of the forty-seven subdepartments (fifty copies each) in all the languages spoken by the staff of DOSE at the time the appeal is written. DOSE will select an unbiased review committee consisting of twenty homeless people from the home state of the complainer, twenty people from each subdepartment of DOSE, and one representative from DOPES who must be from a sport that receives no pay, such as a Pop Warner or AYSO player. The appeals committee must make a decision about the DOPES member's appeal within thirty-six months or have their lunchtime cut to no more than three hours during February, leap years only.

It is expected that the salaries of all DOPES will be raised to (adjusted up or down as necessary) at least GS-1 by the end of five years. This will stabilize sports. However, any of the DOPES not receiving pay for their sport now is prohibited from ever profiting from this legislation. No player of sports or any employee in any position related to sports may profit from any outside activity such as advertising or being spokesperson or mowing lawns or cleaning toilets. DOPES may only receive their salaries from DOSE.

Each DOPES will have three DOSE subdepartment employees to supervise his sports activity and a supervisor for his three supervisors. A user's fee may later be implemented, paid for by each DOPES, not to exceed 120 percent of the DOPES's salary.

The new department will be paid for by a tax on all Americans. The tax is expected to be no more than $1,200 each the first year. Critics are suggesting the tax could be up to $1,200,000 for each family.

All sports fans will be given free tickets to sporting events after qualifying as a sports fan. Also, qualifying sports fans will be free to watch or listen to sporting events for free after purchasing low-cost equipment from DOSE. Only qualified (certified) sports fans will be eligible for events, TV sports, or radio listening. The sporting events will be heavily guarded so no one can illegally learn of the results, thus protecting the rights of the qualified sports fans. All stadiums and fields and even some backyards and patios where some games or contests as soccer or chess might be hidden are expected to be roofed over so no peeping from helicopters or satellites will be possible. Broadcasts of events to fans will be by closed circuit to the special equipment purchased by fans only. Any copying or rebroadcast will be illegal and punishable by imprisonment or death if there is a second offense.

Anyone may easily qualify as a sports fan. Each

applicant for fan status must complete a thirty-one-page application and submit separately a twenty-thousand-word essay about why they want to be a sports fan as the first step. The application and a handling fee must be mailed to DOSE (no checks, credit cards, or debit cards please). Once received, each application will be cataloged and recorded, then reviewed and evaluated in the order received. Each application will be reviewed and approved or rejected by each department of DOSE within five years of receipt. The separate subdepartments will rotate as to which will receive each applicant's submission first. A forty-eighth subdepartment may be necessary to administer this requirement. After and if an applicant has been approved in this first step, a notice to proceed to step 2 is sent to the applicant. There is, of course, to be an appeals process for those people who do not qualify as sports fans, but the details are yet to be worked out by the United States Congress and the Russian Duma. That process will be done within the next decade easily.

The successful fan applicant may then take the notice to proceed to step 2 to the sport club to which he wants to be a fan for approval as a fan of theirs. Each player (DOPES) and his agent must certify under penalty of perjury and threat of legal action that the fan is a decent human being and has never yelled insults, cursed, or beaten up any players or officials of their sport. Once all the players and agents have submitted their certified reports, the fan applicant may take his notice to the stadium or field manager who must certify under penalty of perjury and threat of legal action that the fan applicant has never sneaked into a sporting event without paying or spat on the ground.

If the fan applicant gets all the approvals to date, he may now take his notice to proceed to step 2, etc., to his local cable company, radio, or satellite company for certification that the fan applicant has never copied a broadcast of a sporting event. Once these simple procedures have been completed, the fan applicant may send his notice to proceed to step 2 and his various certifications, along with a certified check of $3,121.22 for processing to the second-step subdepartment of DOSE.

Of course, it is understood that the fan applicant will send along proof of being bonded to the amount of $3,000,000 and insured to the amount of $1,700,000. The subdepartment of DOSE is required to review and process the application quickly. If any fan applicant complains and proves DOSE took more than thirty-six months to process their step 2 application, the subdepartment may be required to work on a Friday sometime in the next year.

When the subdepartment for step 2 (a forty-eighth or forty-ninth subdepartment may be necessary to administer this requirement) has approved a fan's application, his application will be forwarded on to the FBI for clearance. The FBI is required to process the fan application within thirty-six months and return it to DOSE with either approval or disapproval. In such case as disapproval, the fan applicant may be imprisoned until he can prove he is innocent of any wrongdoing. DOSE now sends only approved applications on to the IRS. The IRS is required to review the fan applicant's tax history and report whether he has ever cheated on his taxes or used tax-minimizing strategies over the past twenty-three years. The IRS must report back to DOSE within thirty-six months of receiving the application. Once the IRS has cleared the fan applicant, DOSE will issue the applicant a license to get a fan license.

The fan applicant may take the license to get a fan license to Washington, DC, to the Treasury Department, where a counterfeit-resistant license with the fan's picture, fingerprints, retina print, and DNA clearly visible and embedded in the license will be issued to the now-qualified fan. (A new subdepartment of the Treasury may be necessary to administer this requirement.) A handling fee may be charged to the fan applicant, not to exceed $821.34, by the Treasury Department for their technical work on the license.

The sport fan now may join millions of sports fans and apply for free tickets to sporting events. He may also purchase the special broadcast equipment from DOSE and listen to or view events for free. All sporting event tickets will be free to the fan after he pays the tax of $17.53 and handling fee of $10.13 to DOSE for each ticket. The taxes and handling fees are restricted from being increased to exorbitant rates by this legislation. The legislation allows the taxes and handling fees to increase by no more than 87 percent each year.

For the fan that prefers broadcast sports, he now has the right to purchase the special high-tech equipment from DOSE. The fan may purchase, at cost, radios and televisions from DOSE. The special equipment will not be available from any other source under penalty of mandatory imprisonment for 39.7 years for each violation. The initial cost for a sports radio is expected to be a low $782.71, and for a sports television, a super low $3,180.43 (remotes and color may be available in five years or so). A licensed sports fan, of course, has the right to purchase both a sports radio and a sports television together for a combined price of $4,120.04.

A sports fan may not resell, loan, or transfer his special sports radio or sports television in any way, shape, or form. He may not allow anyone who is not a licensed sports fan to listen to or view his equipment. The special sports equipment can be turned on only by inserting a valid sports fan license into the slot in front of the equipment. When the license is removed, the set is turned off and locked. A sports box microchip uplink to a satellite will detect any tampering or unlawful sports enjoying. (A new satellite may be necessary for this requirement.)

Squads of sport cops will be available for rapid response to any unlawful sports enjoying. Response time for the sports cops is expected to be three minutes or less. (A new law enforcement team may be necessary for this requirement.) Penalties for unlawful sports enjoying will be severe to protect the rights of the licensed sports fan. Any nonlicensed person caught enjoying sports may have all his property confiscated and fired from his job without trial. Decisions to be made by any GS-2 or higher staff of DOSE. (It could be possible that a separate viewing room with security may be necessary for many sports fans that live with a spouse or children or others who are not licensed sports fans.)

Any licensed sports fan who allows a nonlicensed person to enjoy sports on his license will forfeit his sports fan license, undergo horsewhipping in downtown Beverly Hills, and be deported to Pakistan. Appeal processes are, of course, generous as usual. The first appeal will be made to the Ayatollah Khomeini of Iran. Anyone passing the first appeal procedure may then appeal his or her punishment, retroactively only, to DOSE (same procedure as DOPES).

I realize this proposal is far too simple and brief for the federal government to implement as is, so I invite changes and/or additions to get it up to speed. For each change or addition you propose, send $0.02 (2001-dated coins only; no checks, credit cards, or debit cards accepted) to me. Any criticism you send me, please enclose $0.20 (coin only). All funds received will be sent to the Department of Human Services to help them find new ways to withhold pay for citizens' medical care.

CHAPTER 2

The following essays are to critique some of the situations and/or policies of our country.

Our Federal Reserve (Fed) has had a policy of keeping the interest rate very low and much of the time near zero for a good twelve years or more. This action is reportedly to help the economy by making it easier to borrow money and hence start or invest in businesses to grow the economy. I think there are other reasons on the minds of Fed governors and other institutions that have an influence on the Fed's actions but won't be discussed here.

Here, I want to point out some of the harmful effects of the Fed's actions.

Keeping the interest rate very low has made it very

difficult for investors to make a profit for their portfolios and for their retirement accounts. Sure, the policy likely helps people borrowing money, but shouldn't the borrowers pay their own way and not harm someone else? We see lots of news that large pension plans are way underfunded, and it's often implied that the federal government should bail them out of their troubles. It even appears that the federal government may have some contracts that require them to do just that in some instances.

Somewhere in the 1980s, our government encouraged citizens to start putting money aside for their retirement in such things as individual retirement accounts and other types of pension methods that were tax deferred until retirement. The idea was good because it took lots of the responsibility for retirement away from the taxpayer and gave it to the citizen. This makes the retired people much less able to take care of themselves, and government agencies like Social Security and Medicare have way lower ability to meet their obligations. The safety net of Social Security has long been recognized as not enough for most people to live on in comfort, so to supplement one's own retirement is necessary.

To keep interest rates at near zero and often below the inflation rate seems to me to make more people poorer in retirement and more dependent on government largesse. It puts more elderly people on state welfare and more on Medicaid when there is no spare money to pay for extras or emergencies. More housing subsidies, more food stamps, and many other programs to help the needy and elderly have to be expanded, increasing the cost to the taxpayer. Is this the purpose of the Fed, to make us all more dependent on government?

The problem of retirees discussed above isn't the only damage the forced, abnormally low interest rates have done to this country. There is no doubt that the housing crisis we've encountered in the past five or six years was caused by the forced, abnormally low interest rates pushed on us by the Fed. Our cost of houses for several years was rapidly inflated because many people bought houses that they thought they could afford because the interest rate was so low and the house was expected to go up in value faster than our annual inflation. That thinking couldn't be sustained because the houses eventually were not worth the inflated value expected, and the loans became more than the houses were worth. Many people were hurt badly financially by the housing crisis and lost much of their retirement money in the process as they were putting money into their houses that eventually might be sold to supply them some money for retirement. In addition, I know some people who had invested in rental property as a retirement vehicle, and when the drop in housing value hit, they lost their nest egg.

Overall, I think the long time that the interest rate has been kept low has caused more harm to our economy than it has done good for the borrowers of money. It's time to let the interest rate go up or down according to the demands of the economy naturally (supply and demand).

The Fed has also done many things that have greatly increased the inflation rate, such as buying treasury bonds and increasing the money supply. Our federal agencies say the inflation rate is 2 to 3 percent, but just ask anyone buying groceries if it's only 3 percent and you will get a different answer. Sure, many people will switch to a less expensive product when their usual purchase seems to get priced out of their range, but that doesn't change the inflation rate at all.

Price cars and trucks and see if the rate isn't way higher than 3 percent. Many other products are the same. Why does our government obfuscate about that issue? I think it's so our Congress can continue to spend way over their income for favored projects and pay later in inflated dollars. We have a debt of over $16 trillion and no chance of paying it off short of bankruptcy and/or inflation. Either will be a disaster for our economy.

CHAPTER 3

Tax deductions for politicians' favored groups have long been popular in our country. Many deductions might make sense at certain times in history but may not at other times or in different circumstances or amounts. It seems to me that giving money to a charity that has tax-exempt status indirectly costs all taxpayers something in that they will pay more to operate our government when the person deducts and pays less taxes for his donation. I don't object to this in principle, but it has gotten out of hand and taken advantage of in many instances. If someone wants to give to a charity, the money should be all his money and not someone else's duty to then pay more taxes as a consequence.

Big and even huge foundations have been formed over

many years that qualify as charities and have tax exemption. Examples are Ford, Gates, and Rockefeller. Big tax-exempt foundations take huge amounts of money out of the taxable pool. Many of these foundations are worth billions of dollars. One alone is said to be worth $50 billion at its formation. Those $50 billion is now exempt from taxation of its earnings. Let's say that investment of it could earn 10 percent per year, not unreasonable for a capable investment adviser, making $500 million of taxable money. At the current federal tax rate of about 35 percent, this would bring into the United States Treasury $175 million—not an inconsiderable amount. When you add in thousands of other foundations worth many billions of dollars, it becomes big money that is not being due to our government, and that part of the cost shifted to all other taxpayers that don't have tax exemption. Maybe this is part of the reason our Congress and president want to raise taxes for the general public because there isn't enough money coming into the Treasury to run the government the way Congress or the president wants.

Many charitable foundations, some of them university foundations, have been in existence so long and investing their money so long and giving to their recipients so little that they have grown to have such a large amount of money invested that they have influence on the investment market, which may be somewhat unfair to the general public investor. Perhaps some part of the solution to this problem would be to require certain types of charitable foundations to disburse all their money within a given time, such as twenty-five years.

Another thing that annoys me about many of these foundations is that they earned their money in America but give it away to other countries. They can give their money to other countries if they want to, I suppose, but since they are tax exempt in America, as I've discussed above, taxpayers in America indirectly are giving too without any say about it by having to pay more relatively to operate our government. If they want to give their money to foreign countries or foreign people, it should be only their money and not others'.

CHAPTER 4

Recently, I've been seeing complaints about many college graduates not being able to get a job, and some of the discussion indicates there are some degrees that don't have very many jobs available in that category. Some discussions call them worthless degrees. I think any education is better than none, but there may be too many people taking degrees in subjects where there is little need for workers. It seems to me that degrees such as women's studies, African American studies, Hispanic studies, and others may be in that category.

Who then is responsible for those "worthless degrees"? Well, certainly the students majoring in them deserve some blame for choosing a category that may not help them make a living. Perhaps they majored in them, thinking they were easy classes, perhaps for ideological reasons, or perhaps they were counseled to do so by someone.

Many people in this country are too young to remember the late sixties and early seventies when university students were rioting and demonstrating against the Vietnam War. The poor response by the universities in controlling the riots encouraged the students to demand changes and additions in the curricula such as the African American studies, women's studies, and others. I think part of the agenda of the students was to make some easy classes and degrees so they could stay in school longer and avoid the draft and not serve any military service.

Most of the men of the fifties and sixties were required to serve in the military for varied periods of time. Many of the students of the sixties and seventies eventually got advanced degrees of little use except to teach at universities, and that's where they still are perpetuating their jobs by teaching many courses of not much use in earning a living.

The universities deserve most of the credit or blame for those "useless degrees" because they didn't resist the demands or pressure for them. The universities should have recognized they had limited value and held out to award degrees that lead to a profession or gainful employment for most students. Now our children and grandchildren have to deal with taking useless classes while waiting to get into worthwhile required classes.

CHAPTER 5

It's often said our United States is a nation of immigrants. Even first-generation immigrants have often done well. The United States has been a country of opportunity in a world that doesn't appear to welcome hard work or innovation as much. Our recent and present policy doesn't seem to continue keeping the same opportunities open. Now, legal immigrants get help from government in the form of interest-free loans to start businesses such as 7-Eleven stores. I know this sounds like it is a big help to our country too, but this policy helps those less able so we get more immigrants counting on help from the taxpayers instead of immigrants who are able and used to taking care of themselves. I think this is a huge change from previous

US policy and doesn't bring in the same quality of people that we received in years past when success depended on the individual alone.

The US policy takes from the taxpayer to help the immigrants but doesn't really do much for our own citizens. A few years ago, some black people in Southern California had a protest about the Korean immigrants getting help that the black citizens couldn't get. Too bad the federal government didn't pay attention to that message.

CHAPTER 6

I have for some time found it difficult to understand why the foreign policy of the United States should differ from the government policy of China and Russia about radical Muslim terrorist activity. After all, the United States has taken a leadership role in trying to counter terrorism around the world. Yet the United States has criticized both China and Russia when they do something to counter Muslim terrorism in their own countries. At the same time, China and Russia almost always oppose the United States in the United Nations when the United States proposes something to try to counter Muslim terrorism supported by some Muslim countries.

It seems like China and Russia oppose the United States

only to be opposing a perceived enemy even though all countries, especially China and Russia, would benefit and need to cooperate in suppressing Muslim terrorism. As proof, look at the Russian and Chinese support of radical Muslim countries Iran and Syria. Our US diplomats should do a better job of working with two hugely influential countries to get the worldwide terrorist problem under better control. After all, we have a common interest to do so.

The United States isn't exactly consistent in its actions about this problem either. I noticed that all the politicians and officials that commented on the Fort Hood massacre by a fanatic Muslim suicide shooter started their comments by warning not to blame all Muslims so as to avoid retaliation against innocents. I don't say we should do any violence either, but if we always have to stay this politically correct, we allow all Muslims to deny that their religion is largely responsible for the fanatics to continue their terrorist attacks on innocent people. After all, there are actually more Muslim terrorist attacks on their fellow innocent Muslims than on others.

We seldom see or hear of any Muslim leaders condemning a terrorist attack on non-Muslims. They appear to give their tacit approval by their silence. It's true there are many, probably most Muslims, that are not terrorists. But think of the 1930s and 1940s when the "good people" didn't speak up or act to prevent the Nazi terrorists from their crimes. The "good people" of Germany bear some responsibility for what happened there. The resulting World War II to counter the Nazis caused terrible worldwide problems and the death of about fifty million people. So let's not allow the "good Muslims" to have a complete pass for not having the guts or responsibility to speak out against the fanatic Muslim terrorists. I think it would be better for our officials to stop prefacing their discussions about Muslim terrorist attacks with such all-encompassing denials.

I do not understand how the killing of innocent people advances a political or religious agenda or position. It just seems evil to me.

CHAPTER 7

Our national news media, newspapers, and television news have deteriorated over the time I have been interested in the news of the world and news of the United States and even the local news media. Local news usually has exactly the same stories as the other three stations on the same day and at the same times. It appears that world news is only collected by one agency, and all the news channels buy their coverage. I suppose that is economically a good idea for their owners, but it tends to give the viewers only one take on the report given.

That has become more important since the news media have put more opinion into their reports and news stories than previously. I thought that reporting the news by our news collectors was to report unbiased news, but that isn't the case anymore. That appears to be a failure of both the news stations, newspapers, and the journalism schools that have given up on ethics. The "all news all the time" seems to have only two or three stories a day, and they may not be new. There may also be a few nonsense short reports or debates that aren't relevant to the public. Can we ever expect anything from our news media that's pertinent and reliably nonbiased without some kind of outcry that the media will pay attention to? Probably not because it seems that the news is controlled by a small group of people that doesn't care if they tell the truth or not as long as they get their money and get their agenda across.

In the past, I have suggested something a time or two to news media people but have been mostly ignored or put off by them saying that no one was interested in my suggestions, implying that they would do what they pleased with their power. I think that the press has abused that power at times. There have been many times when our very respected newspapers have reported stories leaked to them by traitors to our country that have hurt our national security, but our government won't or can't do anything about it because of "freedom of the press." I think even reporters, newspapers, and TV news stations should be at risk of being charged with treason if they compromise our national security. Of course, there would necessarily have to be some guidelines about that responsibility so the government couldn't abuse the law. I'm sure adequate safeguards could be devised with a little thought.

Sometimes I've thought the constant pounding of one story being reported is being done to distract the general public viewers from other possibly more important things happening. Could that be intentional or just laziness on the part of the news media?

Talking about distracting the public brings up the issue of sports entertainment being so widespread and popular in this country and others. It seems to me that the public should be more interested in the goings-on in the world and especially our own country than in the goings-on in sports or sports players' lives. Why is watching millionaire players play so interesting to so many people? Maybe it allows a lot of people to be lazy and complacent, ignoring much of what is important in the world.

Since we're on the subject of the news media, which is essentially entertainment, I must discuss the entertainment industry as a whole. I have often thought the plots and stories of TV shows and movies are rather narrow and limited in variety. We often see the same plot slightly changed and presented as new. I would like to see more creativity in the new shows and movies as I think we all would benefit.

The writers and producers so often make villains in their plots by putting down our institutions. Scientists, governments, government employees, businesses and its leaders, professionals like doctors and lawyers, military units and commanders, and even presidents and other leaders of countries are ubiquitous in being made villains by the entertainment industry. It's also more common to see the Republican Party made the bad side in any political screed. Even though the technical side of the productions is wonderful, the writing needs to be more varied and creative. Just to prove the point, look at the two movies *Avatar* and *FernGully*, which are antigovernment, antimilitary, anti-business, and even antihuman.

I've almost stopped watching new movies and current TV shows. I've seen all the plots many times. The new movies often are hard to follow when they jump from one time to another and from one part of the story to another without clear transfer. In addition, there is so much background music, noise, and variation in the volume level that I can't hear the entire dialogue. I suggest the writers invent some villains besides the usual because it has become tiresome and sends the wrong message to the children especially.

CHAPTER 8

Paying attention to what's going on in the world should be a priority for responsible adults. One of the important things happening constantly is the actions of the United Nations (UN). Over the years that I've been watching the actions of the UN, there has been a remarkable deterioration in their ability to do the correct thing to improve the world. I have to think that the United States usually has the good of the world in mind when our representatives propose actions at the UN but are so often blocked from the actions advocated by countries' representatives that have far different agendas than to do good for the world—many times blocking actions for their own selfish reasons, but many times just so they can show solidarity with political competitors of the United

States. I see Russia and China veto United States' proposals for no apparent reason. Almost always, some country with poor human rights history is appointed to the human rights committees of the UN. How stupid to expect these human rights abusers to do the right thing in their official duties.

Then there are the corruption and scandals that are pervasive. The responsibilities of the UN are spread to many countries by having people from lots of countries work and maybe in charge of various committees or commissions. Often, those people don't have a tradition of ethics behind them in their countries and favor their friends or inappropriate contractors when carrying out their duties.

A number of years ago, there was so much corruption in one of the commissions that the United States withheld their part of the money to support that commission until the corruption could be stopped. Incredibly, stopping the corruption took several years until the man in charge of that commission could be replaced. The UN officials in charge of appointing the head of the commission were either unwilling or unable to get the corrupt head of the commission out of his powerful position. UN officials largely covered up the issue.

There are other scandals not well covered by the news

media. There have been reports of the UN peacekeepers allowing atrocities to go on when they were supposed to be there to protect people. Then there were some reports of UN peacekeepers' soldiers being part of the problem by being accused of raping some of the people they were supposed to be protecting.

I've seen some suggestions that some of our US military units could be put under the command of the UN. I think that is probably unconstitutional and certainly unwise in light of what I've discussed above.

Because of all the problems of the UN and its history, I have doubts about its ability to solve much of the world's problems and not even its own problems. I think the United States should strongly consider withdrawing from the UN. I think our money that we contribute is a big waste. I think to withdraw from the UN will take several years, so giving notice of the intent to withdraw could give the world and the UN a wake-up call that the withdrawal of the United States would likely be the end of the UN, thus giving them time to correct some of the deficiencies that are so blatant.

Many officials and commentators say we should stay in the UN at least to have a say and some influence, but I think our power is not being used to the best benefit, in fact not being used appropriately at all. The UN and the world love our money, so let's use that power that they have given us.

CHAPTER 9

The technological advances in the United States have benefited almost all of us to some degree. Computers have been a boon in many fields of commerce and other areas of interest. However, computer companies have a long way to go in getting it right. In spite of computer companies bragging that their computers are user-friendly, there are significant problems that frustrate the computer user.

Often, doing some work on a computer takes longer than if we used our older methods of producing the same product. I've seen this many times when I buy something in a store and it takes a long time to complete the purchase when the clerk or cashier has to put in lots more information than they used to when it was only necessary to produce a receipt. The difference seems to be that the store wants to record who is buying and what is sold so their inventory is kept up-to-date. But wait, why should I as a customer have to spend more time and effort for the store's convenience?

Look at the computer operation of our entertainment systems that we all have to program now when in the past all we had to do was turn on one switch. Now I shudder to think about my having to turn on someone else's television when I visit my family or friends, concerned that I will screw up their system. Don't laugh; it's been done to my system several times when I have visitors that want to watch TV when I'm not right there to do it for them.

It should be a scandal for them that computers and software get outdated so quickly. The computer companies and especially software companies stop supporting their products way to soon. That behavior, I suppose, is good for their profit, at least on a short-term basis, but it isn't good for the computer much of the time. It seems to me the best business plan would be to do the best for your customer, and that would be best for the company in the long run too.

I don't understand why businesses have let computer businesses get away with having to get new computers and software so often. Don't think I'm not sophisticated enough to know what I'm talking about because I've been buying computers since the early 1970s and have seen their deficiencies, and they often didn't measure up to what was promised. I didn't and still don't know how to operate computers well, but as an employer for many years, I know what the computer should be doing for me and what it is capable of. Many times, there have been failures to meet my expectations. Talking to others, I have been aware that that thinking is widespread.

Then there is the reliability problem. There are often times when computer systems' reliability fails. I can't name them all, but think of cell phones as an example where often a call is lost, hence not 100 percent reliable. Don't tell me those are phones and not computers because cell phones are largely computers.

Not long ago, I had a cell phone that needed a new rechargeable battery but was otherwise just fine and did all I needed. When I tried to replace the battery, I was laughed at because I expected a piece of equipment I paid for and still worked to be supported by the company that made it. Because of the failure to support the phone by making the batteries for it, I bought from another company. I don't think for a minute that the company I bought from this time will be any better at supporting their equipment because I think there is much collusion between companies for that purpose.

When a company brings out a new version of a computer or software, I have noticed users very often have to take instruction to relearn how to operate the system. I find that a poor tactic by the companies. A user should be able to use the new computer in the same way that he has used his old computer with only learning the new aspects of it. Unfortunately, that's not the case. I've seen users complain that a new version of a software program requires relearning the whole system. I hope computer users will demand improvements in ways that will make computers and software easier to use instead of harder and not require new computers so often. Also, ease of use should be passed on to new software. It is very expensive to replace computers so often for businesses and especially schools. It isn't good for our country to have to spend so much on just that part of their operation.

I recently decided to transfer some of my previously recorded music from cassettes to CDs. When I recorded the cassettes, originally all I had to do was play the music on one device and press one button on the cassette recorder to record the music so I could play the cassette in my car's cassette player. (My current car has no cassette player, hence the need to transfer the music to a CD.) No one-button recording now. To record on a CD, now it requires at least a half-dozen steps, and they must be very precise and coordinated to get the CD right. I don't believe the recording can't be done automatically by the computers of today even easier than years ago on a simple recorder. This is a failure of the computer industry to make a simple job actually simple instead of very complex.

Many other products we use for our personal or business do not require replacing or upgrading so often, such as homes, cars, furniture, radios, televisions, tools, and many others. Come on, Americans; demand the computer businesses do a better job for us.

PART 3

It's time in this book to lighten up the mood, so here are some anecdotes from my own long experience as a physician. Some are funny, and some are not, but still my experience. Names have been changed or omitted.

At the beginning of my senior year at Purdue University, I decided I wanted to go to Indiana University School of Medicine so I submitted an application. Part of the application process was to be interviewed by some physicians. I went to the interview with some apprehension but was put at ease initially by the physicians when they complimented me on my good grades at Purdue in a difficult course of study, biochemistry. They inquired about several aspects of my life at that time; that I was married and expecting my first child to be born in a few months didn't seem to bother them as there were many veterans going to universities at the time on the GI Bill and many were married and had children.

Then they asked me how I expected to pay for medical school. Since I had worked at various jobs during the previous three years at Purdue, I answered confidently that I planned to work part-time during my time at Indiana University too. They both burst out laughing and said derisively, "You can't work and attend medical school because it's so difficult that you won't have time to work." I sheepishly said that I had a little money saved up and that my wife might work.

I went home sure that I had failed the interview. Just before Christmas break, I was surprised to get a letter accepting me to Indiana University Medical School. I did work during the last three years of medical school, and my wife did contribute to the family income. In those days, the state governments were providing about 40 percent plus, I understand, for a public university student's education. I heard the state support of student's education is somewhat less now.

I graduated with no debt except $500 owed to my father for a reliable car to go to my internship out the state when my last junky car blew a transmission during my last month at IU. There were no government-supported student loans available in those days and very few scholarships. I think the interviewers for admission to medical school were looking for students who had the desire, energy, ability, and work experience to finish the course of study.

Anatomy lab was quite stressful in the first semester of medical school as were most of the courses, and the stress was often dealt with by humor. We sometimes had visitors come through the lab while we were working on our cadaver. One time we had advance notice that there were visitors coming. One table of students brought some dried beef to the lab and secreted it within the cadaver. When the visitors came near their table, one of the students pulled a piece of the dried beef from the secreted foil and popped it into his mouth. The visitors were appropriately horrified, and the instructor with them pretended not to see the action.

Our physiology professor was old and set in his ways with no apparent humor, which didn't sit well with some students. The professor would come into the lecture hall and put his three-by-five notes on the table and turn on a flexible arm lamp over the notes. One or two students decided to play a prank, and before class one day, they replaced the bulb in the flex arm lamp with a flashbulb. The professor came in as usual, put his notes under the lamp, and turned it on. The flash was startling and amusing to all the stressed students who burst out laughing. The professor didn't laugh but picked up his notes and left the lecture hall, never to return that day or give that day's lecture, but he still asked a question about it on the next blue book exam. Fortunately, there were lecture notes available on that lecture from the previous years to study.

Our medical school class was made up of very hard workers and excellent students who were used to getting very high grades. The neuroanatomy course was especially difficult. When the first test came along in the first semester, it consisted of pieces of tissue with a nerve in it or a piece of brain with a paper covering all but a small hole in the paper, revealing a tract in the brain for us to identify. Grading was on the curve, and the average for that test was forty-six when we were all used to getting 90 percent and up. This caused a panic in our study time. We were all putting three hours a day in studying outside class time like we had done in undergraduate schools. We all doubled our study time to at least six hours a night because of the test grades, then lied about it to our classmates so they would think they wouldn't have to study so hard to be at the top of the curve in the grading. I think the faculty intentionally graded us low in the early tests to scare us into studying harder, and it worked.

The first two years of medical school were very intense class work and study for hours and hours. It was most intense just before the frequent tests. Several of my classmates and I spent the last half hour or so before each test in the toilet with nervous GI tracts. This problem lasted until our junior year when it became apparent that I was going to make it through the rigorous course of study.

In our junior year of medical school, we were on the obstetrics and gynecology service in a county charity clinic and hospital. The prenatal clinic was a fair-sized room where students supervised by OB residents interviewed and examined pregnant patients in a curtained cubicle with an examining table. There were about a dozen of these cubicles in the room, so there were several students, patients, and supervising residents in the room at any one time.

One of my classmates was interviewing a pregnant patient before examining her. In the interview, it was revealed that this was her sixth child and she was not married. Being at a time when moral questions were still queried routinely, my classmate asked the patient how she got pregnant when she wasn't married. She became indignant and reached into her purse, pulled out a photo of a man in a sailor's uniform, pointed at the photo, and said in a very loud voice, heard throughout the clinic, "See that, see that son-of-a bitch? He told me he was sterile." This, not surprisingly, stopped all the other activity in the clinic for a few minutes while everyone laughed. The poor lady left in a huff. Nowadays I expect no one would dare ask how a patient got pregnant when she wasn't married.

The obstetrics service gave us a social education besides medical training. We students were required to stay with a patient in labor all through the labor and delivery no matter how long it took. One of my OB patients was a twelve-year-old girl. She did pretty well during the whole labor time under my supervision and counseling, but I was floored when we took her into the delivery room and put her legs on the stirrups for the delivery and she asked me why. When I told her it was so we could deliver the baby, she said, "Through that little hole?"

Another twelve-year-old obstetrics patient was asked by one of our female students how she came to be pregnant. The little girl replied that the seventh grade had a Christmas party, with no further comment.

After a long and traumatic labor, constantly calling to the student doctor "Help me, Doctor, help me, Doctor," the patient was finally delivered of the baby and her labor pains relieved. She then said, "Thank you, God."

In our third and fourth years, we spent most of our time in clinics and hospitals with professors and residents in hands-on learning. We still had two hours of lectures each day at lunchtime when we could eat while listening or take notes and skip lunch. During the lecture series on surgery, a student on the surgery service at the time was required to present a surgery case that he was involved with to the professor and chairman of the department of surgery (Dr. S.). The presentation was always stressful for the student presenting because the professor was pretty volatile. He also was a stickler for demanding knowledge about the history of the type of surgery being discussed at the time and often grilled the class on the history.

When my turn came to present my case, I was about twenty minutes early, so I spent the time in the library looking up the history of that type of surgery, including the pioneers that did the first cases. The professor showed up on time. I presented the case and stood by at the lectern expecting the professor to grill the class on the case and the history. Instead, the professor started asking me the history. I answered every question and must have looked very knowledgeable. He asked me everything that I had looked up in the library in about twenty minutes, and I knew nothing more. At that time, he was called back to surgery for an emergency, saving me from revealing my ignorance.

While interning in the US Army, I experienced some interesting things. Fort Knox was a basic training facility in the 1960s. At the five-hundred-bed hospital at Fort Knox, Kentucky, I was assigned to the medical ward. I arrived one morning to have the charge nurse tell me that I had a new patient, just arrived a few minutes ago, in bed, such and such. I went to see him immediately. He was an eighteen-year-old recruit. He had a brand-new plaster cast on his arm. I asked him why he was on the medical ward instead of the orthopedic ward. He told me that he had just arrived on post during the previous night from an Ohio recruiting station on the bus. He had been vomiting all the way to Kentucky and even in the barracks. A sergeant saw him vomiting and ordered him to go on sick call. Since he was late for sick call, he ran across the base to get to sick call on time, but when he jumped across a little gully, he fell and injured his arm. At sick call, he was x-rayed and a minor fracture of the wrist was found, then he was placed in a cast and sent to my ward to find out why he was vomiting and to treat him.

I took his history and found that he had just graduated from high school a few days before coming to Fort Knox and had been a football star at the school. He said that he always vomited before every football game because he was nervous about the game. Now he said he was nervous about his new life in the army and thought he was vomiting because of that. I checked him over thoroughly and found no physical cause for the vomiting, and he had no more vomiting while in my care. I concluded that he was only vomiting from his nerves as he thought. I sent him back to duty for his basic training. I often wondered what his mother thought when she heard that he had a broken arm and was hospitalized in less than twenty-four hours of joining the army.

I had another vomiting soldier at Fort Knox too. He also got admitted to my medical ward direct from sick call. When I took his history, I asked how long he had been vomiting. He said, "About a year." This was surprising to me, so I asked why he was just now being admitted to the hospital for it. He said that he had been vomiting in the latrine every morning for months, but that morning, the sergeant saw him and ordered him to go on sick call, where he was ordered into the hospital. Not knowing what was wrong with him, I did a very extensive workup and evaluation of him as the vomiting over such a long time could be very serious. I got consults from various specialists, but the diagnosis was obscure until I had the psychiatrist see him. The psychiatrist said he was psychotic and transferred him to Walter Reed Army Hospital for boarding out of the army. All kinds of people got inducted into the army in those days.

After four years of ROTC, four years of reserve service while in medical school, and a year of active duty as an intern, the army sent me to Fort Sam, Houston, Texas, for "orientation to the army." The temporary duty assignment (TDY) was for five weeks. It was easy duty as it consisted of mostly lectures and a little field duty of camping and firing weapons. The students were all young doctors, dentists, and veterinarians who were to serve their duty right after the "orientation." All were, of course, recent university graduates. At least 90 percent had at least some ROTC, and many of us had interned in the army. That made us all already very familiar with the functioning of the army, thus making the lectures very boring and repetitive.

We were even marched from place to place by some second lieutenants fresh out of college even though we were all captains at the time. That of course didn't go over too well with either the lieutenants or the captains. We mostly knew the contents of the lectures and spent the time in them to either read novels or medical literature when the lights were on or sleep when the lights were off to show slides. After all, we mostly had just finished eight years of intensive study and a year or more of extremely busy internships and residencies, making the "orientation" a much-desired vacation.

One of the long lectures was about the number and types of aircraft in various army units. The lecturer showed slides in the darkened hall, allowing many of us to doze off. All of a sudden, the lights came on, and the lecturer called out "All right, you there, Captain" and pointed to a doctor near the front, apparently discovered sleeping. "Stand up, how many aircraft in an army division?" The doctor stood up warily and, after about a minute, said, "Ah, a bunch." All of us, now wide awake, burst out laughing as no one could have kept up with the number of aircraft listed even if we had been paying attention. The colonel, who was lecturing, said "You got the idea" and then continued the lecture.

Fort Sam was a nice needed vacation. We were able to take our families and even had all evenings and weekends free to be with them—new to us at the time. I had a nice apartment with a swimming pool where my two kids, aged two and four, learned to swim in those five weeks. Also on weekends, we explored the area.

The Cuban nuclear missile crisis was in 1962 while I was at Fort Knox in an ear, nose, and throat (ENT) fellowship. When the crisis came up, a friend, Dr. C., in the same fellowship was pulled out of that duty to be assigned to a tank battalion. I continued in the ENT fellowship because I was assigned to Fort Ord Hospital but on TDY to Fort Knox, and apparently, Fort Ord was not on alert for the crisis.

My friend Dr. C. had to be available to ship out to Cuba in only two or three hours' notice and in the meantime was expected to put together a medical unit of personnel and equipment to serve the tank battalion in case they went to Cuba and engaged in battle. The tank battalion prepared to go by preparing and loading their tanks on railroad flatcars with all equipment and personnel packed and ready at an hour's or so notice. The battalion never went to Cuba that time, but I always had a healthy respect for the preparedness of our military after that. I, of course, did extra duty while Dr. C. was off doing the battalion surgeon job. That was only the first experience of me having to double up on duty when other doctors were pulled off their usual duty and sent elsewhere. When I finished the ENT fellowship and arrived at Fort Ord, I was assigned to the ENT clinic every day for eight hours, the emergency room for two nights a week, first surgery call one or two nights a week, and ENT call most nights as there was only one other ENT doctor. I was very busy, of course, but I had a nice duplex within a few minutes from the hospital. When the Vietnam War escalated in late 1963, my duty was expanded to take sick call at a dispensary and run a sixty-bed pneumonia ward before clinic hours. Needless to say, I was very, very busy and decided not to stay in the army when my obligation was up. I am proud to say, however, that all that responsibility and work prepared me to be a better family physician for the rest of my career. The work definitely helped my maturity as a physician.

There were a number of interesting things that happened during my duty at Fort Ord. I was working with a fully trained ENT doctor (Dr. N.) there, so I got a lot more experience in ENT, but the army sent Dr. N. to the House Clinic in Los Angeles for six months to learn to do stapedectomy, which was new at the time. A stapedectomy is a surgical procedure to restore hearing loss due to middle ear bones and joints getting frozen and not moving properly. That, of course, left me to run the clinic by myself, making even more work. Fortunately, it was before the Vietnam escalation, so I could handle it.

There were a lot of retired military people in the area of Monterey and Pacific Grove, so we often saw them and their families that were eligible. One of the retired general's wives often came to Dr. N. for any cold or sinus problem. She would walk in ahead of all the recruits waiting in line and announce to our sergeant that she was Mrs. General S. and needed to see Dr. N. He would see her, of course, as that was the army culture. While he was away in Los Angeles, she came in and did the usual announcement. The sergeant told her that Dr. N. was away for several months and that Captain Johnson was the only doctor on duty in the ENT clinic until Dr. N. got back from TDY. She agreed to see me then as she knew me a little from my being present when she came in a few times before.

When I looked at her, she had a broken nose that was way off to the side of where it belonged. I asked what happened. She said she had bumped into a door. I had heard that many times before when a person had been socked in the face and had something broken, but I didn't question her further, just assumed that the general had popped her. I told her that she needed to have the nose put back in position by general anesthesia and a doctor, and

I suggested that I would do it the next day. She refused and said she wanted Dr. N. to do it. I said she shouldn't wait more than a few days or she would have to have a rhinoplasty to rebreak the nose after it has healed a bit. She still didn't want me to do it.

I guess a captain wasn't high ranked enough as Dr. N. was a major. There were also several ENT doctors in Monterey that she could go to, so I didn't push it. I thought it was funny but went over to the surgery unit and told the chief of the surgery department about her and asked if he wanted to fix her nose as he was a colonel. He laughed and said, "No way, Clyde, that's your job."

A few days later, Mrs. General S. came back to the clinic and told me she was ready to let me fix her nose. I figured she had by then seen a private ENT or so and didn't want to pay the price, or she trusted the army more. After all, I had by then fixed lots of broken noses working at bases where there were lots of fights among the basic-training soldiers. I took her to surgery the next day and set her nose with no trouble. She came back a week later for recheck, and the nose was in perfect position. She found out when Dr. N. was back and came to see him for his opinion and approval. I never saw General S. the whole time. That's one of the reasons I concluded that he had slugged her. She was a very pretty woman of about fifty years old.

Another army experience has to be told too. At Fort Knox, the officers' club automatically sent all officers a monthly bill, which I paid even though I seldom had time or inclination to use. I just paid it because I knew the army officer culture. Two of my fellow interns had no idea of the army culture as they were graduates of Loma Linda University, who had no ROTC program. Because of religious reasons, they also didn't want to be around where any drinking of alcohol was done, and of course, that's mostly what is done at the officers' club.

Consequently, the two young doctors didn't pay their officers' club dues. Officers not paying bills are strongly frowned upon by the army, so that act got reported to the general of the post, Fort Knox. The general called the two doctors in to his office and gave them an army ass chewing. They were naive and objected on religious grounds, but the general made them pay up to the time that they saw him and exempted them for the rest of the time at Fort Knox.

I was aware of that incident when I went to Fort Ord. I expected the officers' club to automatically send me a bill. Since I had no time to go to the club anyway, I thought nothing of it until I received a letter from the officers' club at the end of the year 1963 telling me that they didn't have my application on file and to send them another one that they enclosed. Since I was getting released from active duty in another four months or so, I just laughed and tossed the letter and application in the circular file.

A week or so later, I got the same letter through channels, which means it went through all my superiors, like the hospital commander and the department of surgery, etc. You can't ignore a letter sent through channels, so I took the letter to the hospital commander's office and asked the warrant officer who essentially ran the office what to do about it. I said I didn't use the club as I didn't have time or desire to drink. He said to just say that and send it back through channels, which I did.

A few days later, another letter through channels came, wanting me to certify that I had never used the club. I did so and sent the letter back through channels again, expecting that to be the end of the matter. But it was not to be. A few days after, the warrant officer from the hospital commander's office came to my clinic and said that the hospital commander (Colonel B.) and I were to see the past commanding general (Major General T.) about the officers' club issue and set up a date and time for the meet. Wow, that was momentous as I seldom saw the hospital commander and never the post commanding general. Knowing the army culture well by then, I was of course apprehensive about it.

The day came, and Colonel B. and I, along with another doctor, Captain K., stood at attention in front of General T. He gave us a long lecture about esprit de corps and related subjects for a good fifteen minutes. He then asked if we had anything to say for ourselves. Poor Captain K. said yes—he had joined the army to get some training and experience but instead had been sent to Korea to serve in a dispensary and then at Fort Ord in another dispensary where he saw little besides common colds and then felt it not right to make him join the officers' club. General T. interrupted angrily then and said "No one is making you join the officers' club" and continued the ass chewing for another ten minutes or so.

The general then turned to me and asked if I had anything to say. I said, "No, sir." Then Colonel B. said the same, and we were dismissed. I walked across the post back to the hospital and entered through the dental clinic door. There I met a dentist that I slightly knew who committed that he heard that I had to go see the general. Yeah right, no one was making us join the officers' club, ha. I bet there wasn't another officer on the post that didn't join the officers' club that year. I'm not exactly proud of that incident. I knew better than to challenge the army officer's culture.

The emergency room at the Fort Ord five-hundred-bed hospital was very busy. It was not unusual for two doctors and several WACs and corpsmen to see and treat over a hundred patients a night. The enlisted corpsmen and WACs were quite well trained and were very helpful.

One night, after an unusually busy session, I had just got to lie down in the call room at about 2:00 a.m. when the corpsman came in and asked me to come and see a patient. We never turned down a patient's request to be seen, so I got up. The patient was the wife of a private, who showed me a burn on her finger, which was an obvious cigarette burn that was mildly inflamed. I asked how long since she burned it, as it looked intentional. She said she burned it over a week ago. I wondered then why she was just now getting it treated. She said she worked. I ordered her treatment but felt that after a full day's work in my clinic, running the sixty-bed pneumonia ward before my clinic, and then another intense nine hours working at the emergency room that she and her husband, who was with her, had abused the right to use the emergency room and my patience.

Since the emergency room record had the soldier's unit

listed, I asked the corpsman for the unit commander's phone number. The corpsman enthusiastically looked it up, and I dialed the number. It was for a Lieutenant W. I heard a sleepy hello on the line. I told him that this was Captain Johnson at the hospital emergency room. He quickly answered, "Yes, sir, what is it?" I told him about the soldier's misusing the emergency room at 2:00 a.m. for a nonemergency and gave the soldier's name. He said he would take care of it right away. I couldn't get to sleep the rest of the night. I felt so guilty, but the corpsmen were real happy.

I did over a thousand tonsillectomies at Fort Ord, both under general anesthesia and under local anesthesia. That included children dependents and soldiers who had needed it before joining the army and got sick frequently because of chronic tonsillitis. In those days, that was the treatment for recurring problems with the tonsils.

For a month we had a surgery resident who wanted to get experience in ENT, so I supervised him doing a tonsillectomy. It looked like the procedure went well, but of course, I couldn't see into the soldier's mouth very well.

The procedure was finished, and we left the operating room. I went to the clinic, but the resident doctor went to lunch. I soon got a frantic call from the recovery room that the young soldier was bleeding badly from the mouth. I ordered him back to surgery and rushed over. The resident couldn't be found. With the soldier lying on the operating table, coughing up and spitting blood, filling a basin quickly, the nurse anesthetist, Major Ann M., said, "Oh shit, the last one of these I had died."

I tried to reassure the soldier after that, but he sure still looked scared. I told the anesthetist to intubate him so I could stop the bleeding. That nurse was so good that she put him under and intubated him through all the blood in about three seconds. After that, it was easy for me to tie off the bleeder. The nurse anesthetist surely saved that soldier's life, not me so much. He was later pretty grateful. I only wish the anesthetist had had more tact.

All officers at Fort Ord were required to go to the firing range and fire a weapon, usually the .45 pistol. A group of officers from the hospital went to the range together when ordered to do so. The enlisted range officer was happy to tease officers about their poor shooting even when they were doctors who were not expected to do any shooting in a war. However, I got some respect when he announced over the loudspeaker that the officers there that day should go over to the eye, ear, nose, and throat clinic to have Captain Johnson there help them see better to shoot as he was the only one from the hospital who qualified on the .45 pistol. I had long ago fired expert on the M1 and the .22 rifles in ROTC summer camp.

Fort Ord personnel also supported the Hunter Liggett Military Reservation, sixty miles or so south of Fort Ord, where a lot of training and maneuvers were done. A doctor was stationed there to take sick call. When he went on leave, a doctor from Fort Ord was sent there to fill in until he returned to duty. The hospital commander asked for volunteers to go to Hunter Liggett for a week at a time. It looked like easy duty to me, so I volunteered to get a little time off from my usual extremely busy schedule.

The duty there was actually very light, and I only worked about two hours a day. One night while I was there, I was called out for an auto accident that a soldier had nearby. He was severely injured, and it was obvious he needed to be in the hospital for surgery. The officer of the day agreed, and the soldier and I were air evacuated by helicopter to the Fort Ord Hospital. Riding the helicopter was quite the experience. One of the old missions was only a few hundred yards from my barracks, so I spent some of my free time learning some mission history from the priest there.

The year 1964 saw the Vietnam War rapidly escalating, so I was discouraged from staying in the army where I would be sent to a combat zone. I had done my share of sacrifice for my country by being associated with the army for eleven years. I left the army and joined the only family doctor (Dr. E.) in a small town in Idaho. We had a primary clinic and a small hospital in the county seat and three outlying clinics in smaller towns, twenty to thirty miles away in all directions.

A few weeks after joining Dr. E., he asked me to go to one of the towns where we had a clinic to be present during the annual rodeo. A doctor and an ambulance were required to be at the rodeo to take care of any injuries. I was happy to go as I had never been to a rodeo. Johnny, the ambulance driver / lab tech / x-ray tech, and I were sitting on the ambulance hood next to the rodeo gate on the evening of the rodeo. The first event to open the competitions was a bull rider, a bronc rider, and a bareback rider all at the same time. As you can imagine, there was lots of action.

When the dust cleared, all the animals were out of the arena, but the bull rider was lying on the ground writhing in pain, clutching his shoulder. Johnny and I put him on the gurney and into the ambulance. He said his name was Super S. and was a local cowboy. I examined Super and told him I thought he had a dislocated shoulder and that we would have to take him to our hospital for an x-ray to confirm it and reduce the dislocation, then x-ray it again to be certain there was no other problem with the shoulder.

The hospital was twenty-five miles away over a curvy, mountainous road. Super, thinking of the difficulty getting to the hospital, said, "But, Doc, they'll have to stop the rodeo until we get back and that will take at least two hours. Just give me a shot and fix it, I trust you, I'm sure you're right." Well, since I was young and knew everything and just out of the army and had done everything, I said, "OK, I'll try it."

Actually, a dislocated shoulder is best treated very soon after injury, before swelling occurs, to block the reduction. I gave him a shot of Demerol IV to relieve the pain and muscle spasm. Within about two minutes, I was able to slip the shoulder back into place. Once the dislocation is reduced, the pain and spasm is gone. Super stood up, swinging his arm around, and announced he was fine. I told him he must keep the arm in a sling for a couple of weeks to allow the ligaments to heal and that I still needed an x-ray to be sure there were no fractures or chips of the bone. He promised to come to our clinic the next day for the x-ray, then walked off to get a shot of something more, I think. He never came for the x-ray, and I never saw him again. Those cowboys are tough.

During another rodeo, a bull rider came to the office with a back injury after being thrown from a bull. An x-ray showed a fracture of a transverse process of a vertebra in the lower back. I put him in a brace and prescribed pain medications even though he obviously had already drank something for pain. He said he planned to ride a bull again in that evening's events. I strongly advised against that but later heard that he had done just that.

Another rodeo incident was when Dr. E. went to a rodeo about forty miles away where we had another of our outlying clinics near the Salmon River. During the events, a steer roping team was competing. The steers are several hundred pounds and moving rapidly away from the ropers. One of the cowboy ropers got a loop of rope around his thumb at the same time he got the rope around the steer. When the steer fell, the rope put tremendous pressure on the cowboy's thumb and amputated it at the hand. This happened in the 1960s, so there was no grafting the thumb back on.

One Friday evening, I received a call from the hospital to go see a forest service employee. He had been out in the national forest doing hiking trail work all week. Early in the week, he had fallen and cut his hand. Since he was walking alone and had planned certain trail work for the week, he used some fishing line and sewed up the laceration and bandaged it. He continued the trail improvement work he had planned the rest of the week and got back in town that Friday evening and thought he should have me check his wound. The wound was slightly infected but was healing well, and the sutures he had put in with fishing line were holding the skin of his palm together well. All I could do was compliment him on his ingenuity and treat the minor infection.

One of the young nurses told me she was uncomfortable catheterizing men when there was no man in the little hospital to do it, especially when she knew almost everyone in town. She was able to get past the concern after I told her she was a professional and the men would understand that about her if she projected that attitude.

A mother brought her eight-year-old into our main clinic and frantically related the problem that the child had swallowed a nickel-sized slug from an electrical box. An x-ray showed the slug caught in the trachea but not obstructing the breathing much at the time. I had no instruments to go down the trachea after it and also felt I didn't have the experience either. I quickly loaded her and the boy into our flying club's airplane (a 4-place Stinson 108) and flew them to the Boise Airport where we were met by an ambulance and taken to the hospital there where an anesthesiologist removed the slug from the boy's trachea.

Flying in Idaho was common, and I did a lot, but not enough to stay proficient apparently. I planned to fly the Stinson cross-country to Denver to take a continuing education course. I had my wife and three of my four children along. The day was stormy and windy. As I landed in Rock Springs, Wyoming, for fuel in a strong crosswind, the wind picked up the big Stinson wing and dragged the opposite wing on the ground. That is called a ground loop. No one was injured, but the wing was damaged, and we had to take the train on to Denver. Our mechanic flew the Stinson back to Boise for repairs.

I wrecked another airplane a little later. It was wintertime and not much to do, so on a free afternoon, I volunteered to take the local veterinarian for a ride in our flying club's Cessna 150. As we did the takeoff run down the runway, I couldn't keep the plane going straight down the runway, and we ran it into the snowbank made when the snow was plowed off the runway. The propeller was damaged. I think my friend, the veterinarian, was tense and braced his foot on one of the ailerons on his side, so I couldn't guide the plane with the ailerons on my side of the plane. I lost my confidence in my flying after that and didn't fly much even for the patients.

Providing medical care to a tough rural population can be very challenging. In the fall is hunting season in Idaho when all the male citizens and some of the females go hunting no matter what. One of my usual patients came in with a swollen ankle from a stumble at his ranch. An x-ray revealed a fracture that I put in a walking cast. This was before fiberglass casts were invented, so it was a plaster cast. As I was wrapping the plaster, the patient said to me, "You better make that cast real strong because hunting season opens tomorrow." I told him it wasn't a good idea to go hunting then with the cast on as he would still have some pain and swelling, and if the cast got wet, it would get soft and ineffective, letting the walker break off. Sure enough, he came back on Monday, two days later, for a new cast after walking in snow hunting deer and elk. The next weekend, he went hunting on horseback.

One of my patients, a forty-year-old lady, became pregnant again after having four miscarriages. She was very worried about possibly miscarrying again and wanted the baby very badly. She came to our outlying clinic thirty miles from our hospital and clinic and lived in a fairly remote area. I saw her every week during the whole nine months for checkup and reassurance.

Just when she was about due to deliver, she came to the weekly visit crying uncontrollably. I was worried that something was wrong with her pregnancy. After I got her calmed down enough to find out what was wrong, she told me she felt fine. The problem was, she had found out that a family who lived up the canyon from her had a child die the night before, and she was sad because she wanted a child so bad. The family up the canyon didn't believe in medical care and did not seek care for their child with a sore throat and a fever. She said this was the second child that family had let die. My patient soon delivered a healthy baby boy.

I expected the modern West of the 1960s to be pretty tame, but it was not to be in Idaho. One day about noon, as I was about to leave our main clinic for lunch, a man walked in the door with blood all over his head, shirt, and even on his pants. This patient eventually led to my first time to testify in court for a patient. The story came out over a short period of time about this mini range war.

My patient was a sheepman. He was Basque and had a ranch and leased range from the BLM and Forest Service to graze thousands of sheep. The day he came in to my clinic all bloody, he and his Basque sheepherders had gone to his range and found a neighbor's cattle on his range. He ordered his men to chase the cattle off his range and onto the cattleman's range. About that time, the cattleman and his cowboys rode up. There was some dispute and shots were fired, but no one was hit. Nevertheless, the boss of the cowboys and the sheepman both came off their horses and beat each other over the head with rocks.

My patient had twenty-five or so lacerations on his head requiring sutures, along with other bruises and abrasions over his body. Apparently, the cattleman had much the same injuries but had gone to another town with a doctor farther away. The sheepherders and the other cowboys seemed to have avoided any injuries. My patient was hospitalized for several days to recover.

In those days, it was possible to recover from relatively minor injuries and illnesses as the cost was not nearly as high as now, and the rules for such were much relaxed and under my decision instead of an insurance company. I went to court in another town to testify about my patient's injuries. I heard some of the testimony of the Basque sheepherders but could not understand it as they spoke only Basque of their native Spain. The final decision of the court didn't resolve much as it was concluded the two injured shared the blame for the encounter. That was my experience with a range war, however small.

There was other violence around too. In one of the small towns we serviced, a deputy sheriff got into an argument with a cowboy in the local bar. There were bars in all the small towns but not many other services. The cowboy left the bar but came back a few minutes later with his gun and shot the deputy dead. All these things happened in only three years that I spent in Idaho.

An old rancher was brought by his wife into my clinic in a wheelchair after he fell from his horse during roundup. When he saw me for the first time, he gave me a dirty look and growled, "I thought you had to graduate from high school before you could be a doctor." His wife said to him, "Now be nice." I later received a quarter of beef from them. Not only did we eat plenty of beef there but also had venison, elk, bear, duck, and trout to eat frequently.

I eventually had to leave Idaho because the economy of the area could not support two doctors. I moved to California where I had lots of other interesting experiences.

In addition to my family medical practice in California, I was medical director of a nursing home for over twenty-five years and had many elderly patients. Sometimes there were funny incidents such as the time a little confused Pop

E. wheeled himself up to the nurses' station where there was a small turtle in a little aquarium. He reached in, grabbed the turtle, and swallowed before the nurse could stop him. We monitored him closely for several days, but he had no ill effects. Pop E. also wasn't totally confused as he sometimes wheeled up behind a nurse bending over attending to a patient and put his hand up the nurse's dress. This was some time ago when nurses still wore dresses instead of pants.

Another time, Pop wheeled up next to the nurses' station and next to a lady patient also in a wheelchair. He quickly put his hand up the lady patient's dress. The nurse saw that and quickly removed Pop's hand and told him to stop that. The lady patient, known to be a little confused too, said to the nurse, "He wasn't doing anything wrong."

A ninety-year-old man (Mr. R.) came into the office and told my receptionist he wanted to see the doctor. She asked him what his problem was to start our evaluation. He said, "I need something for my nature." The receptionist and medical assistant were stumped as to what he wanted, so they couldn't prepare him for me in advance. When I saw him and asked what was wrong, he said there were a few widows who came to see him sometimes so he needed something for his nature. I got the message and gave him a testosterone shot. This was before Viagra was invented. Every three months or so, Mr. R. came back for another shot of testosterone, apparently doing well and keeping the widows happy.

After a couple of years, Mr. R. became a little confused and unable to care for himself, so I admitted him to the nursing home. One day after he had been there a while and not getting his testosterone shot anymore, as I came into the door of the nursing home to see my patients, the nurse met me, all excited, and said, "What are we to do? We just found Mr. R. in bed with Mrs. J., and they weren't sleeping either." I said, "Pull the drape around the bed." I thought it best they have some privacy.

Another of my nursing home patients was an ex-nurse with a loud voice and pretty healthy but unable to walk very well. Her 107th birthday came up, so we planned a party for her. The local newspaper sent a photographer. He asked her to what did she attribute her long life. She loudly said, "I think it is because I never got married." The whole roomful of people laughed and didn't dispute her reasoning.

It seems like the nursing home was undergoing almost constant surveys and inspections from one agency or another. Falls, broken bones, and bedsores were frequent problems that were monitored. Untrained officials were often complaining about patients being restrained to prevent injury but then really citing the facility when a patient wasn't restrained well and suffered an injury, making it damned if you did and damned if you didn't.

As the medical director of the facility, I was constantly watching for dangerous things that might result in an injury to patients. A day or so after a fire inspector was in the facility doing a survey, I noticed a latch in the middle of the hallway floor for a fire door to close onto during a fire. The latch protruded about an inch above the smooth hall floor, making what I thought was a hazard for elderly patients walking the hall and often dragging their feet. Tripping on this latch could easily cause a fall and a broken hip in the frail elderly patient. I discussed the hazard with the administrator, who of course was very concerned that it could cause a preventable injury. Workmen set the latch deeper into the floor soon after my reporting it. About a year or so later, I noticed when walking in the hall that the latch was again protruding. I asked the administrator what was going on. He said the fire inspector made them change the latch back, never mind the hazard to the patients. I gave up the effort. You can't beat city hall. The fire inspectors were more powerful than real safety issues.

One of my areas of expertise was treating industrial

injuries. For many years I was the physician for glass manufacturing companies on job injuries. They ran three eight-hour shifts a day, so I often got called at night to treat an injury. Most of the injuries were minor cuts and burns. I lived much closer to my office than my partners, who were a surgeon and a cardiologist, so I had to take the night calls for these industrial injuries, but also partly because the safety officer for the manufacturer wanted me to do most of the medical care for their employees.

I could get to my office in about five minutes in the middle of the night, but often, the patient, also five minutes away, would not arrive for another thirty to forty-five minutes. Annoyed about waiting that long, I would ask what took so long. The patient invariably said he had stopped at the bar on the way for a drink. I guess that put me in my place and showed what was more important to the patient. It wasn't getting medical care.

There is an interesting story about this glass manufacturer that closed many years ago too. At the time, I was paying my trained medical assistants the going rate of about $3.50 per hour. The glass manufacturer was paying the union member women packing their bottles $6.10 per hour, no training required. The union went on strike to get more pay for the women. The union won more pay, but the manufacturer went out of business soon after as they could not compete with the cheaper plastic containers. Many of the glass company's employees remained my patients, and it was notable that many could not find a job of any kind after that.

Another of my industrial clients was the company making the huge tunnel for the Feather River Project, bringing water from the Feather River in Northern California to Los Angeles. An entrance to that tunnel was close to my office. Companies often took me on plant or site visits to see what type of injuries I might encounter in serving their employees. The drilling company did also, so I was taken down a deep hole where we got on a full-size train to go into the tunnel where the drilling was done by a huge drilling machine, and the premanufactured concrete pipes were placed right behind the drilling machine. Apparently, this was a smaller version of a drill that made the Chunnel from France to England. I also was taken to an area far up the mountain where the same company was building the generator in the same project. These site visits, among several others, gave me insight into lots of manufacturing and construction, so I felt I was able to do a better job.

For about a third of my career, I tried to do the full range of family medicine, including obstetrics. Eventually, I had to give up obstetrics because my partners weren't trained to do obstetrics and the insurance got too expensive for me to continue. One of my regular families came in once, the mother and her eighteen-year-old daughter. The daughter was having abdominal cramps that were said to be very severe. When she lay on the examining table and I exposed her abdomen to examine her, it became obvious what was causing the cramps. The full-term pregnant uterus stood up in a major contraction. I quickly transferred her to the hospital delivery suite where I delivered her of a baby boy to the surprise of both the mother and daughter.

Another surprise came one day in the office when my very competent cardiologist partner (Dr. M.) came to my side of the office and excitedly pulled me into an examining room where he was seeing a young woman in terminal labor. There was no time to transfer this patient to the hospital delivery suite, so I delivered the healthy baby girl right then in the office.

Speaking of delivering babies, way back in the 1960s, it was unusual to allow fathers or anyone into the delivery room to observe the delivery. In the small town in Idaho, it was unheard of until I started allowing it for selected fathers. Some fathers didn't want anything to do with seeing their wives going through the pain of delivering a baby. Later when it became much more common for fathers to observe and even participate to some degree, the fathers began to be pressured to be there by their wives and by the acceptance of the practice in general. I'm afraid some of the fathers aren't too happy to be in the delivery room after all.

There is lots of moviemaking going on around my California practice. One day a number of years ago, one of the cowboy stuntmen came into my office from a couple of blocks away where he was working with horses for movie stunt work. He had been thrown off a horse and hit his head on the corral fence and had his scalp ripped half off his head, exposing the white skull. I was surprised there wasn't much bleeding seen after I cleaned up the wound, being it was a scalp injury that usually bleeds heavily. After seeing the extent of the scalping, I advised that I have the surgeon come in and do the repair in the operating room even though all the tissue was still there. The patient, being a tough cowboy, refused and wanted me to just sew up the scalp. I injected the scalp with local anesthetic, pulled the scalp back into place, and sutured it in place without any problem—much easier than I thought it would be. A week later, when I took out the sutures, it was healed well.

I had other movie industry patients from time to time. A director brought a very beautiful actress into the office after she had wrecked a jeep in a scene being filmed for one of the popular TV shows. She had severe pain and spasm in her back. An x-ray showed spasm but no fractures. This was before CT scans and MRI scans were available. I gave her pain relief and prescriptions for pain. The director was livid that I wouldn't inject her back and send her back to work right away. He said he had hundreds of people waiting and it was costing him thousands of dollars not to have her on the set filming that day. I didn't give in, though, as I was more sympathetic to the young woman's pain in her back.

Even without the lack of empathy for the actress, I've not been very anxious to provide care for industrial injuries for the movie companies. Many times, there were problems getting paid for my work. The usual ploy not to pay was, "He wasn't working for us that day, so we're not responsible." We couldn't then get the patient to decide who was responsible to pay either. I didn't seek business from the movie companies because this was a frequent ploy.

My partner Dr. T. did sometimes make agreements with a TV company to rent out parts of our office or his small hospital for filming an episode of a TV show. An episode of a popular show about two motorcycle policemen was filmed at the entrance to the hospital. It took most of the day. I didn't get much done because all the nurses, medical assistants, other female workers, and even patients were too busy watching the handsome actors. I had to do all the work myself.

Another time, the star of a detective show was filmed walking into our office door. That didn't take all day, but our young x-ray technician was a patient in the small hospital at the rear at the time and was very upset that she didn't get to see her hero, the star, in person. One of the front office girls told the star when he was in the office, so he walked all the way back through the clinic to the hospital to the tech's room and gave her a kiss to get well. Needless to say, that made her day.

A bit later on, I had occasion to see more of movies and TV shows being made locally around our area. It's surprising how many and how long it takes to film a few minutes of action. The quality of the shows is without equal, and I can see why in the meticulous way the filming is done. When I watch the show, however, I sometimes wonder why we don't get the high quality of writing to match the technical level.

Our private office practice often had patients that were primarily drug seekers. Many drug users were welfare patients. Drug addicts and heavy drug users can't hold a job, so they are on welfare and Medicaid. Since we saw lots of Medicaid patients, we had lots of drug seekers. Once a drug user has convinced a doctor that he needs the drug, it's hard for a doctor to end the relationship with the patient. After all, physicians are trained to try to relieve pain and suffering too.

Dr. T. was seeing one of his regular patients in one of our outlying offices when he became a little suspicious that he might be an addict because he was in to get his narcotic prescription so often. Dr. T. had his medical assistant watch out the window when this patient had an appointment. Even though this patient was on welfare and Medicaid, he arrived in a limousine and left in a limousine with another man in the passenger seat waiting in the limo for him. The conclusion was that the patient was able to get narcotic prescriptions because of his medical condition but was likely selling all or at least part of the medication to a drug dealer. Dr. T. refused to see that patient again, but likely, the patient would be able to convince another doctor he needed the narcotics. This and other reasons, it is very difficult to stop drug abuse in this country.

I had a man come into my office wanting me to become his physician, he said. He had a beautiful copy of a medical history showing he had tic douloureux (a condition of severe pain in the face), with consults from a neurologist, and that he needed Dilaudid in such heavy doses that I would have to see him weekly and write a lot of narcotic prescriptions, about double my usual number. Dilaudid is a very strong and addicting narcotic. After all, I had never used Dilaudid in my practice in my whole career. I thought that would draw scrutiny from the Drug Enforcement Administration (DEA).

The records were from a hospital in the east of the country. I didn't like the idea that I would just be a drug supplier for this patient and was also suspicious of the records he had. I suggested he go to a neurologist that usually handled that type of problem, and then I told him I didn't want to take his case. I was even more suspicious of the records not being his and that he was just another addict when he became irate about the refusal to take him as a patient, and stomped out of the office. He demanded to get his money back, indicating that he had paid cash in advance. He had no insurance, and expected to get his drugs just by paying an office fee and getting no exam or evaluation. There was no chance of that in my office.

I hope these stories have been as entertaining to you as they were to me as they happened.

www.ingramcontent.com/pod-product-compliance
Lightning Source LLC
Chambersburg PA
CBHW032016170526
45157CB00002B/729